Luna Lotus

CHAIR YOGA

for seniors

OVER 60

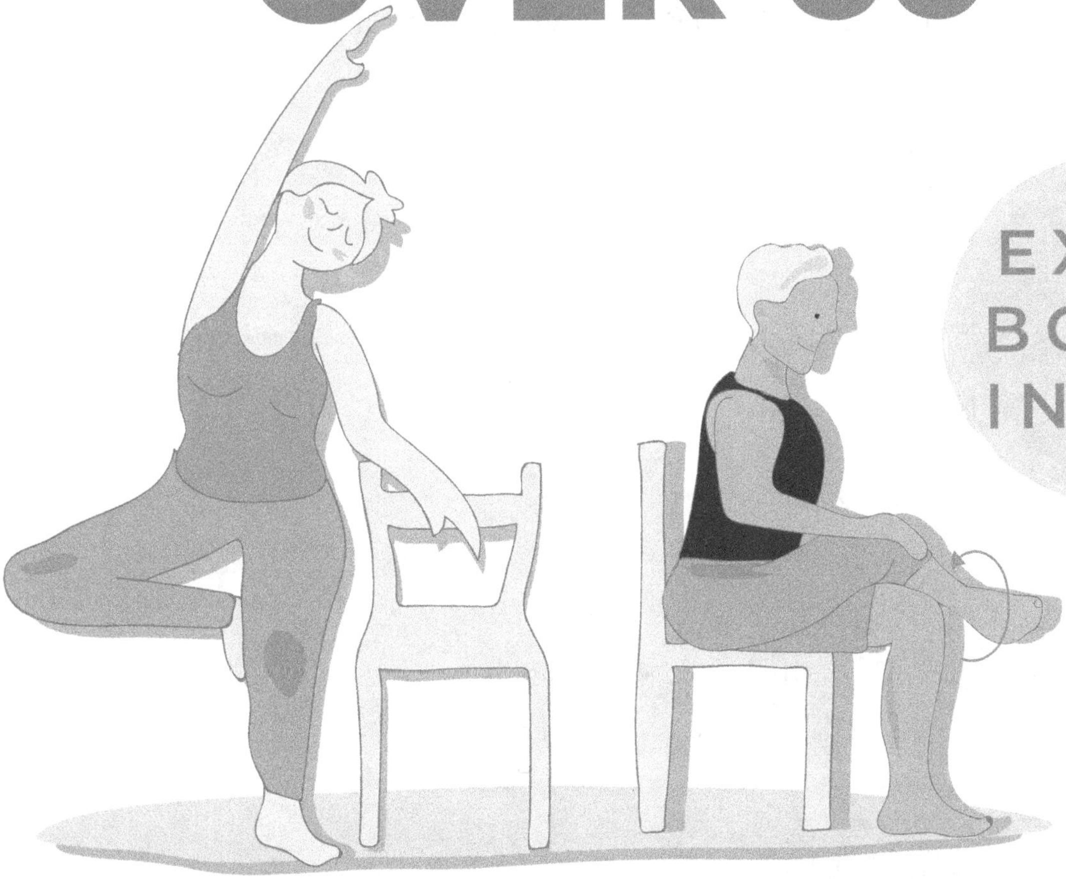

EXTRA BONUS INSIDE

GENTLE EXERCISE
TO REVITALIZE MIND & BODY

This book is dedicated to everyone who knows that aging is not a reason to give up and let yourself go, but rather a reminder to invest in your potential and to strive towards attainable goals through persistent effort.

"May the guidance within these pages inspire you to keep pushing forward and to never give up on the possibilities that await you, no matter your age."

Luna Lotus

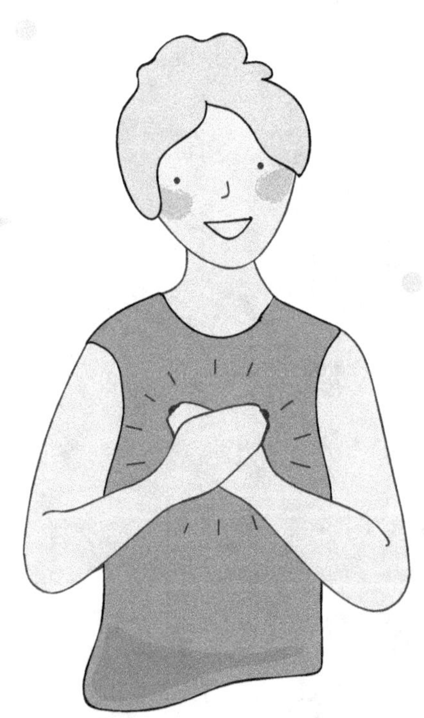

CHAIR
YOGA
FOR SENIORS

EXTRA BONUS

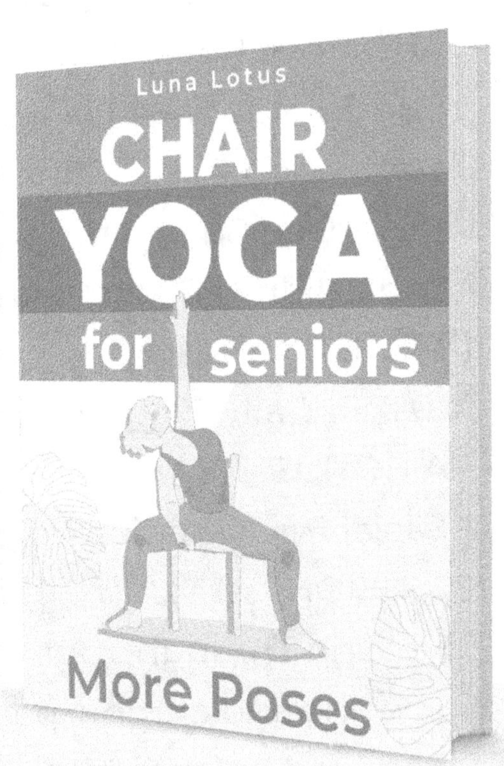

Your support means a lot to me and would be invaluable in spreading the word about my work.

If you enjoy this book, please consider leaving a review!

www.yoga.flyedition.com

Table of Contents

THIS BOOK BELONGS TO

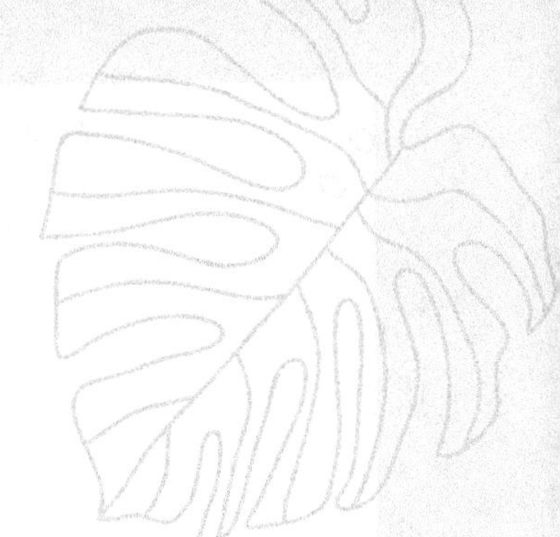

Name ....

Date ....

Your Commitment to a Better You:

....

....

....

A MUST-KNOW FOR YOUR WELL-BEING

"Motivation is what gets you started. The secret to achieving your goals is perseverance".

INTRODUCTION - The Seven Chakras

The chakras are energy centers along the spine that are important in yoga and meditation. They relate to a variety of facets of our health, including both physical and spiritual.

◈ The root chakra (Muladhara) symbolizes our connection to the earth and is related to feelings of security, stability, and grounding.

◈ The sacral chakra (Svadhisthana) is linked to feelings, connections, and interpersonal relationships.

◈ The solar plexus chakra (Manipura) is associated with self-confidence, and the capacity to come to conclusions and make choices. It is also linked to metabolism and digestion.

◈ The heart chakra (Anahata) is the center of love and compassion associated with forgiveness.

◈ The throat chakra (Vishuddha) is associated with communication and creativity and is connected to the thyroid gland which regulates metabolism.

◈ The third eye chakra (Ajna) is linked to intuition, perception, and the pineal gland which regulates sleep.

◈ The crown chakra (Sahasrara) represents our connection to higher consciousness. It is associated with spiritual awakening, inner peace, and enlightenment.

Each chakra is associated with different aspects of our emotional, physical, and spiritual well-being. When our chakras are balanced and flowing freely, we experience optimal vitality and health. For example, if we have a blocked or underactive root chakra, we may experience feelings of insecurity or lack of grounding, while an overactive third-eye chakra may result in excessive daydreaming or difficulty focusing. Balancing and opening the chakras can be achieved through various practices such as

◈ Yoga: a physical and mental practice that combines poses (asanas), breathing exercises (pranayama), and meditation to improve overall health and well-being.

◈ Meditation: a technique that teaches the mind to acquire calmness, clarity, and relaxation.

◈ Sound therapy: a therapeutic approach that promotes healing and relaxation through sound vibrations produced by instruments such as singing bowls, gongs, chimes, or tuning forks. Sound therapy has significant health advantages that have been demonstrated.

◈ Aromatherapy: a holistic therapy that uses plant extracts and essential oils to promote physical, emotional, and spiritual well-being, often through inhaling or applying the oils topically.

These practices help activate and balance the energy in each chakra, promoting a sense of harmony and well-being. You can also focus on specific yoga poses or meditation techniques that target each chakra to open them and promote healing. With regular practice and attention to these energy centers, you can cultivate a deeper understanding of your own body, mind, and spirit, and enhance your overall well-being.

So, next time you practice yoga or meditation, pay attention to these energy centers and see how they can help you on your journey of self-discovery and well-being.

"By understanding and balancing the energy in each chakra, you can promote physical health, emotional balance, and spiritual growth."

The Main Types of Yoga

There are numerous variations of yoga, each with a special focus and methodology. The most popular varieties of yoga include:

- Hatha Yoga: It is a style of yoga that emphasizes fundamental poses and controlled breathing techniques. It is characterized by a gentle and soothing approach, often used as an introduction to yoga for beginners.

- Vinyasa Yoga: It emphasizes flowing movements that are synchronized with breathing. It can be quite challenging and dynamic, with each movement flowing seamlessly into the next.

- Ashtanga Yoga: It is a type of yoga that is more challenging in terms of physical exertion and follows a predetermined series of postures that are executed in a particular sequence.

- Iyengar Yoga: It is focused on precise alignment and incorporates various accessories, such as blocks, straps, and blankets, to support practitioners in achieving proper alignment and posture during their practice.

- Kundalini Yoga: This is a more spiritual form of yoga that emphasizes meditation, breathing exercises, and chanting. It is thought to stimulate the energy located at the lower end of the spinal column and bring about spiritual transformation.

- Bikram Yoga: Commonly referred to as hot yoga, this type of yoga takes place in a heated environment to induce sweating to eliminate toxins and enhance flexibility.

- Restorative Yoga: This relaxing form of yoga uses cushions like bolsters and blankets as props to help the body relax into meditative positions for an extended period of time.

"These are only a handful of the numerous types of yoga that exist. Each type of yoga has its unique benefits and can be tailored to meet your specific needs and capabilities."

Are you having difficulty picking up things from the floor or experiencing back pain?

Do you also struggle with mobility or balance issues? Feeling stressed or anxious? Are you looking for exercises to stay active and healthy as you age?

This was me, I can relate to how you feel. My life was sinking, and I had lost my energy and enthusiasm until I discovered chair yoga.

"Don't let physical limitations stop you from enjoying life. Chair yoga can help you!"

◈ Chair yoga is a safe and effective way to improve your health gently, without having to get down on the floor or strain your body.

What You Need to Start

To practice yoga on a chair, you will need:

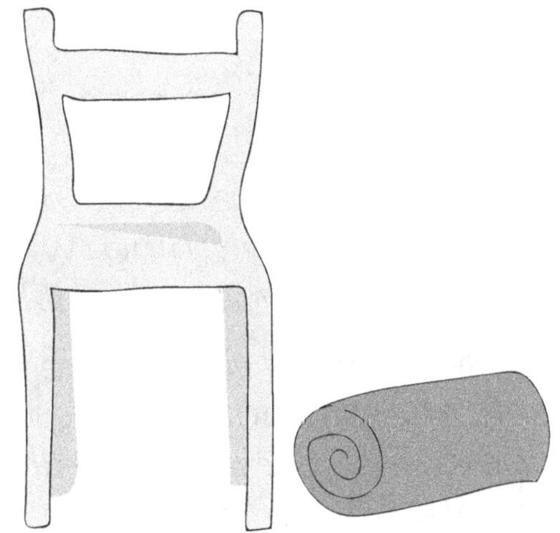

◈ a sturdy chair without wheels,

◈ comfortable clothing,

◈ a towel to roll up and use as thickness.

Make sure that you have a safe, clear and uncluttered space to practice.

Finally, you will need an open and willing mindset, ready to explore the benefits of yoga from the comfort of a chair!

Chair Yoga Benefits

Did you know that chair yoga has the same benefits as traditional yoga and is even more powerful?

◈ *The seated position helps to keep your back straight, avoiding the stress of standing positions, and makes the exercises for the back, arms, and neck more effective.*

◈ *The seated position also doesn't stress the knee and ankle joints, which can be under pressure during seated floor positions. Balancing exercises can be practiced with eyes closed on a chair, eliminating the need for torso twists when practicing the same exercises standing with the support of a wall.*

◈ *Sitting comfortably in a chair, all concentration is focused on the exercise and breathing to avoid falling. Chair yoga is exceptional for seniors, but it is suitable for all ages!*

Did you know that yoga goes beyond simple physical activity?

◈ *It is a multifaceted approach to wellbeing that considers the mind, body, and spirit.*

◈ *One of the most important aspects of yoga is conscious breathing, which can have incredible benefits for your overall health and well-being.*

◈ *When we're born, we breathe naturally and effortlessly, but as we grow older, our breathing patterns become shallow and erratic, often centered in the chest causing tension and blockages in our chakras.*

This is where yoga breathing exercises, also known as pranayama, can be incredibly powerful.

So, welcome to chair yoga!

This book is designed to help seniors experience the benefits of yoga without having to get up and down from the floor.

With chair yoga, your body undergoes changes that improve your ability to perform daily activities like bending, stretching, getting dressed, taking a bath, and moving around the house safely, which leads to ***happier days and the freedom to spend quality time with your loved ones,*** without constant pain and limitations.

As we age, our bodies go through changes that can make daily activities difficult or even impossible to perform. You may overcome these restrictions and keep your mobility and freedom by practicing chair yoga.

Chair yoga is like a warm and cozy hug for your body, mind, and spirit! It's a special type of yoga perfect for everyone, no matter your age or physical capabilities.

With the support of a chair, you can explore gentle stretches, soothing breathing exercises, and easy movements that make you feel good from the inside out.

The best part about chair yoga is that it encourages you to be kind to yourself and honor your body's needs.

You don't have to push your limits or contort yourself into difficult positions – you can simply relax, breathe, and enjoy the moment. This helps reduce anxiety and stress and increases your overall sense of well-being.

When you practice chair yoga regularly, you will notice that you feel more relaxed, calm, and happy. You will even experience physical benefits like improved flexibility, balance, and strength. Plus, you will feel more connected to the world around you and to yourself.

Just remember that everyone's body is different, so it's important to listen to your body and adjust the practice to your needs. And if you have any medical concerns or limitations, you should consult your doctor before beginning any new workout program.

So, grab a chair and let's start exploring the wonderful world of chair yoga together!

BREATHING EXERCISES - PRANAYAMA

Before starting any chair yoga poses, it's important to begin with a few minutes of conscious breathing.

And the best part is that you can practice these breathing exercises anywhere, anytime – whether it's in bed, on the couch, or during a break.

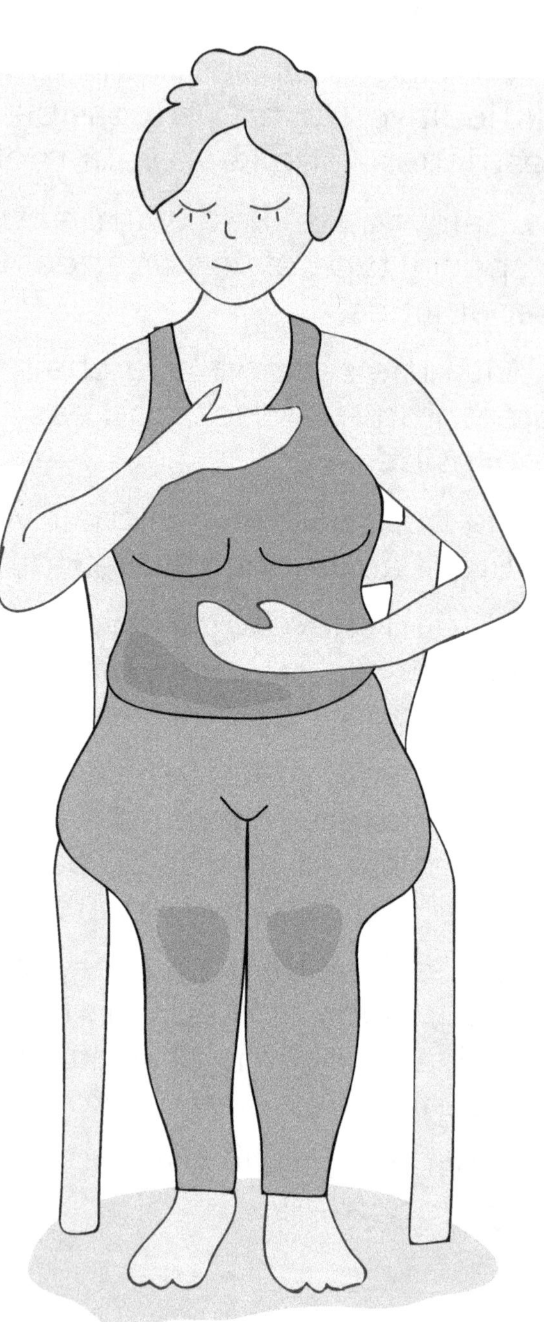

"By making conscious breathing a part of your daily routine, you can transform your breathing habits and improve your overall health and well-being."

Calming Breathing

◈ Start with your back straight in a relaxed position.

◈ Gently place one hand on your chest and the other on your belly, to evaluate your breathing.

◈ Relax your body and mind and take a few normal breaths.

Diaphragmatic Breathing

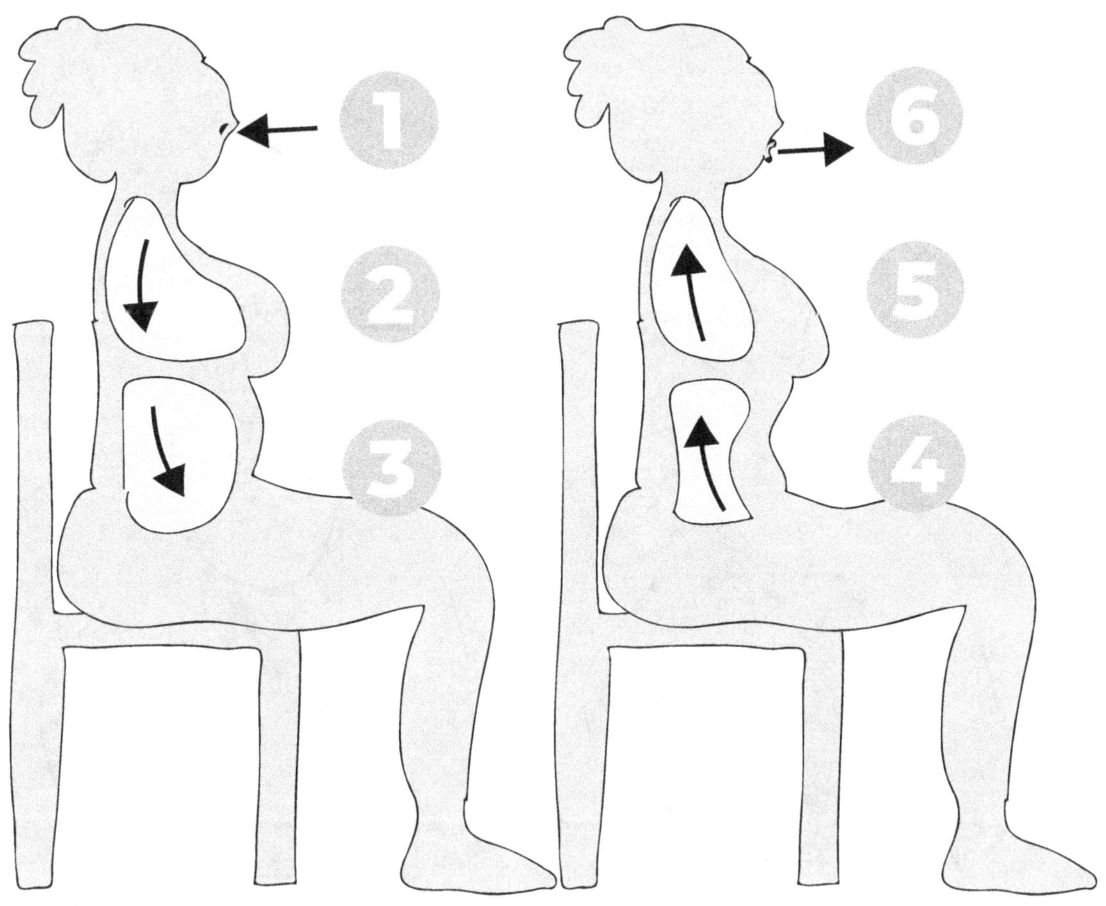

◈ Start with your back straight in a relaxed position.

◈ Place one hand on your chest and the other on your belly to assess your breathing, making sure to do so gently (see previous image).

◈ Take a few deep breaths through your nose to relax your body and mind.

◈ Inhale through your nose while mentally counting 4 seconds and in the following order, make your chest inflate, then your stomach, and finally your belly like a balloon.

◈ Exhale through your mouth while mentally counting 6 seconds emptying your belly, stomach, and chest.

◈ Repeat this cycle of inhaling for 4 seconds and exhaling for 6 seconds several times.

◈ Then take a few normal breaths to relax.

Alternate Nostril Breathing

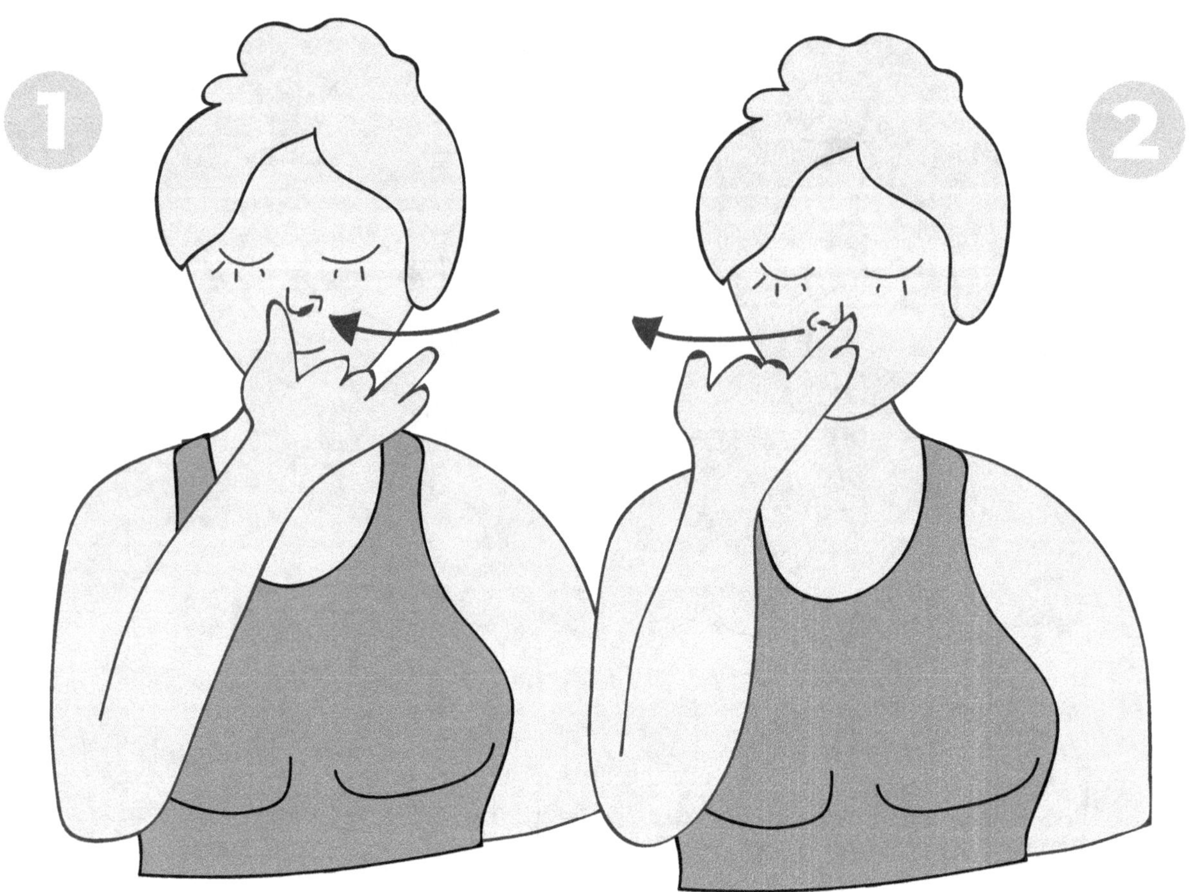

◈ Gently shut your right nostril using your right thumb, while taking a deep breath through your left nostril.

◈ Seal your right nostril with the right ring finger and exhale through your right nostril.

◈ Deeply inhale through your right nostril, then, while releasing your left nostril, seal it once more with your thumb.

◈ Completely exhale through your left nostril, then inhale through the same nostril while sealing it with your ring finger.

◈ At the same time release your right nostril.

◈ Continue alternating nostrils in this way for a few rounds, inhaling and exhaling deeply through each nostril.

◈ When you are ready to finish, complete the cycle with an exhalation through the left nostril and then release your hand on your knee, breathing normally for a few moments.

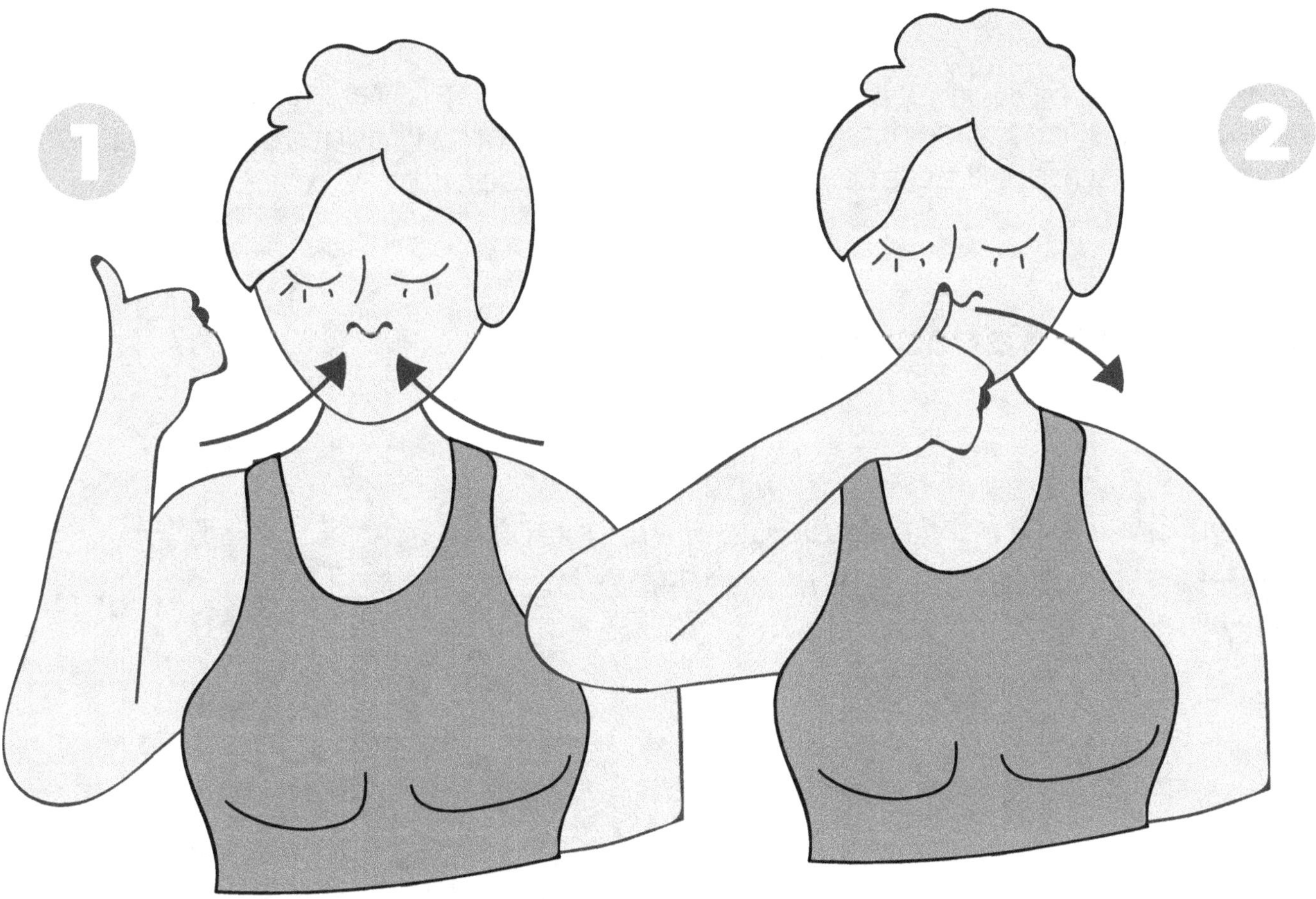

◈ Deeply inhale with both your nostrils.

◈ With your right thumb, shut your right nostril.

◈ Completely exhale through your left nostril.

◈ Then inhale again through both nostrils.

◈ Repeat this cycle for a few times.

◈ Then take a few normal breaths to relax your body and mind.

"Don't give up on your journey and keep striving to become the best version of yourself."

LIGHT POSES 'GETTING BACK ON YOUR FEET'

A daily session of gentle exercises to improve balance, flexibility, breathing, and concentration, ideal for seniors who have undergone an operation, suffered an accident, or with a disability.

Chair Pose Tadasana

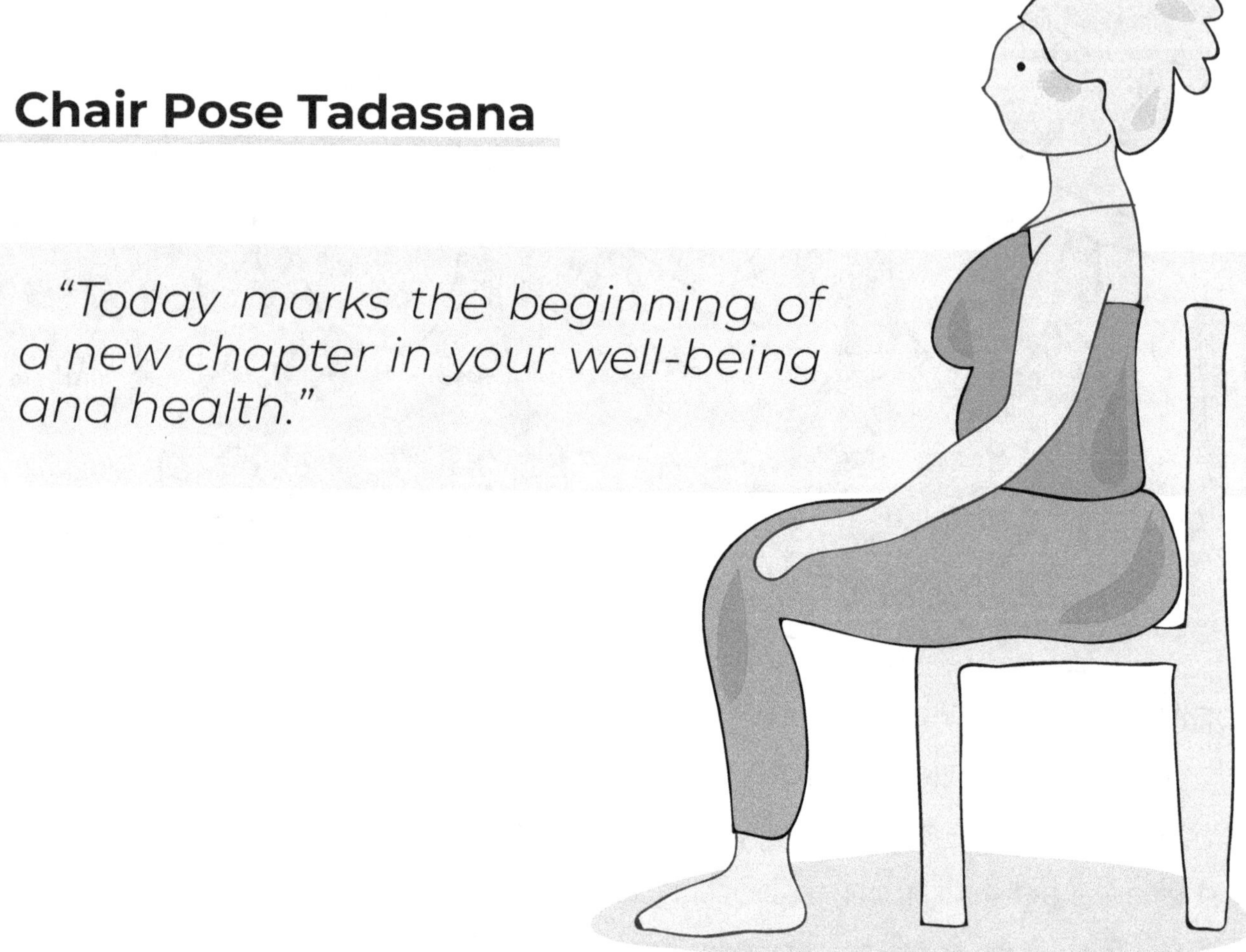

"Today marks the beginning of a new chapter in your well-being and health."

◈ Sit up with your back straight, hands resting on your legs, your feet flat on the ground.

◈ Hold this pose for a few breaths, focusing on your alignment while breathing deeply.

Relieve your back pain, improve your posture, build your strength, and find inner peace with this pose.

Half Moon Right and Left - Neck Rolls

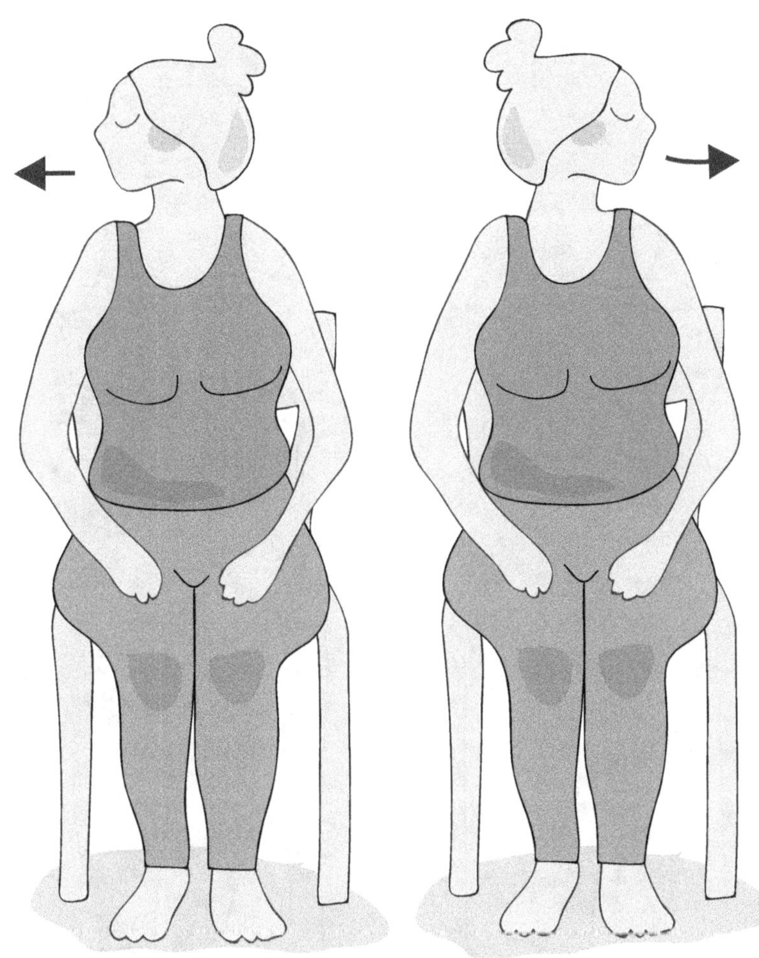

◈ Relax in the chair with your back straight, your hands resting on your thighs, shoulders relaxed.

◈ Inhale and during exhalation turn your head to the side and hold it for a few seconds.

◈ Inhale and return your head to the center.

◈ Repeat by turning your head to the opposite side.

While breathing in and out, repeat several times.

This helps relieve back pain, improve posture, and relieve neck and shoulder pain.

Half Moon Up and Down - Neck Rolls

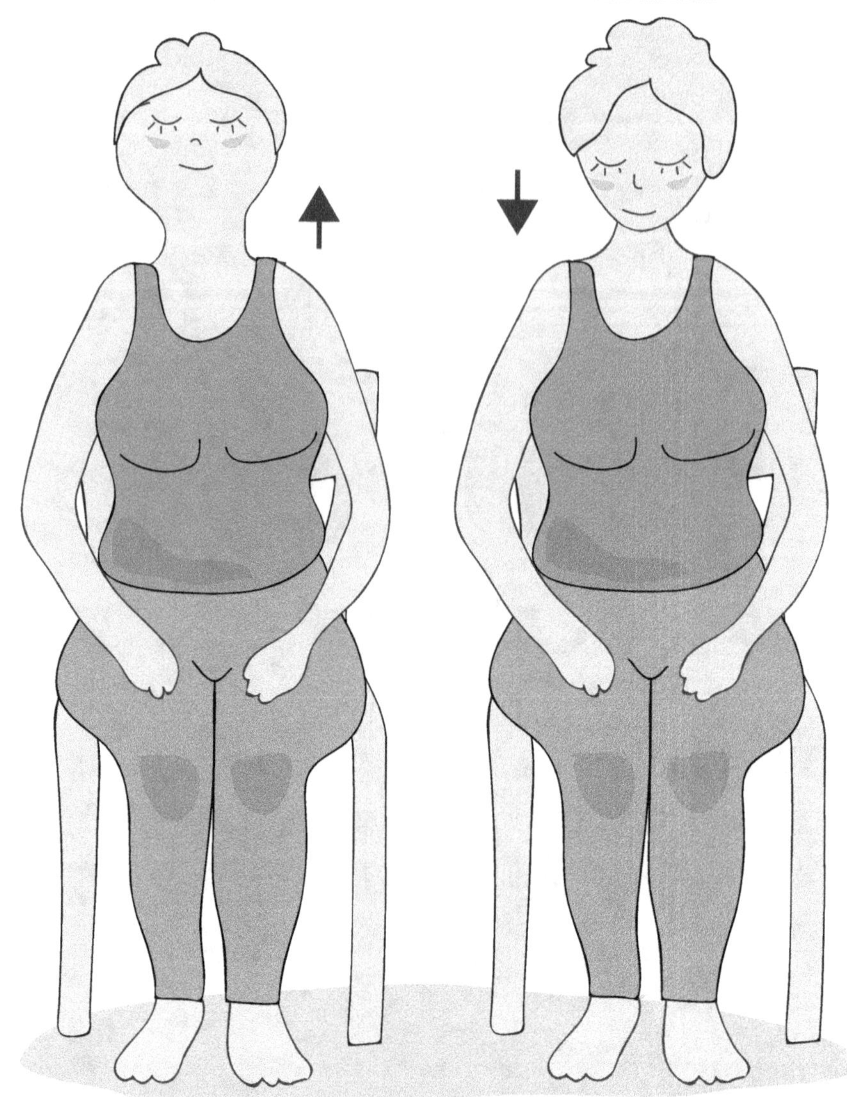

- ◈ Exhale and gently lower your chin towards your chest, stretching your neck.

- ◈ Inhale and rotate your head backward, bringing your gaze towards the ceiling.

- ◈ Continue to perform the upward and downward movement in a slow, controlled motion for a few breaths.

- ◈ On your last exhalation, bring your head back to the center and rest for a moment before repeating the exercise.

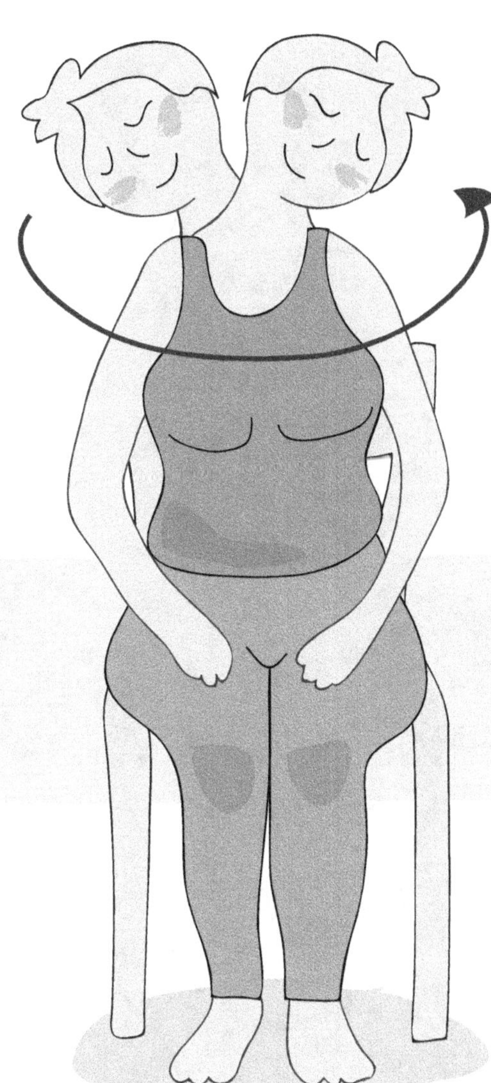

"It's time to begin your journey towards a stronger and more vibrant you."

◈ Inhale and gently lower your chin towards your shoulder, then start rolling your head back and then to your left ear.

◈ Exhale and continue rolling your head bringing your chin towards your chest.

◈ Continue to roll your neck in a slow, controlled circular motion.

◈ Repeat the circular motion several times in one direction, then change and rotate in the opposite direction.

◈ On your last exhalation, bring your head back to the center and rest for a moment before moving on to another exercise.

Handhold

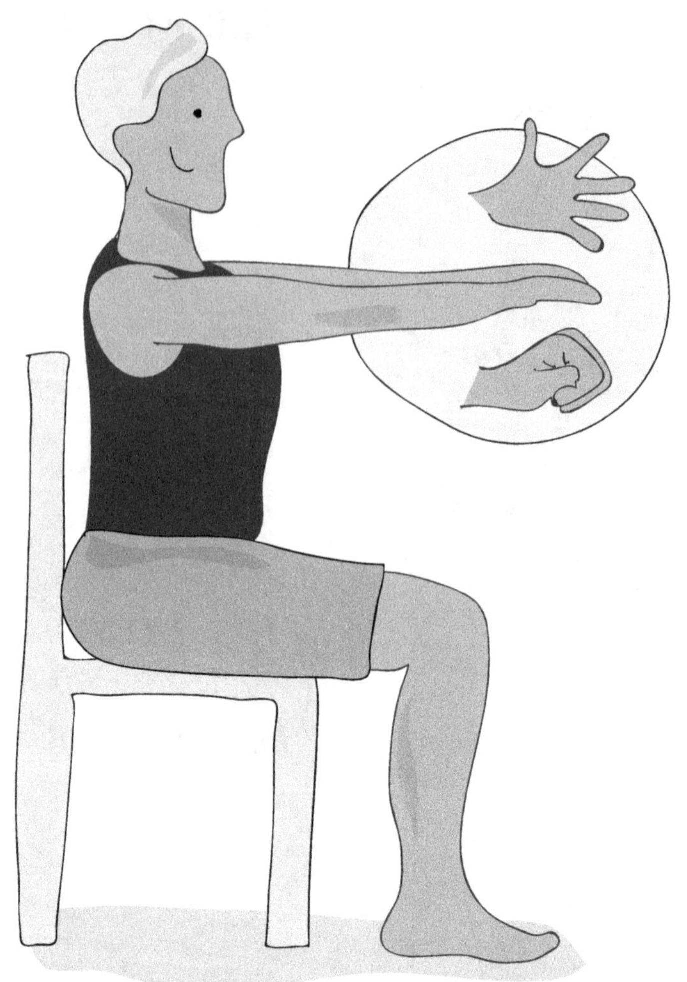

◈ Raise your arms horizontally.

◈ Inhale and spread your fingers apart, stretching them as far as you can.

◈ Keep the posture for a few seconds, feeling the tension in your hands and forearms.

◈ Exhale and slowly make fists with your hands, squeezing them tightly.

◈ Feel the tightness in your hands and forearms while maintaining your fist for a short period of time.

◈ Inhale and release your fists, extending your fingers again.

Repeat the exercise several times, moving slowly.

This helps to reduce tension in your forearms and hands and to strengthen your grip.

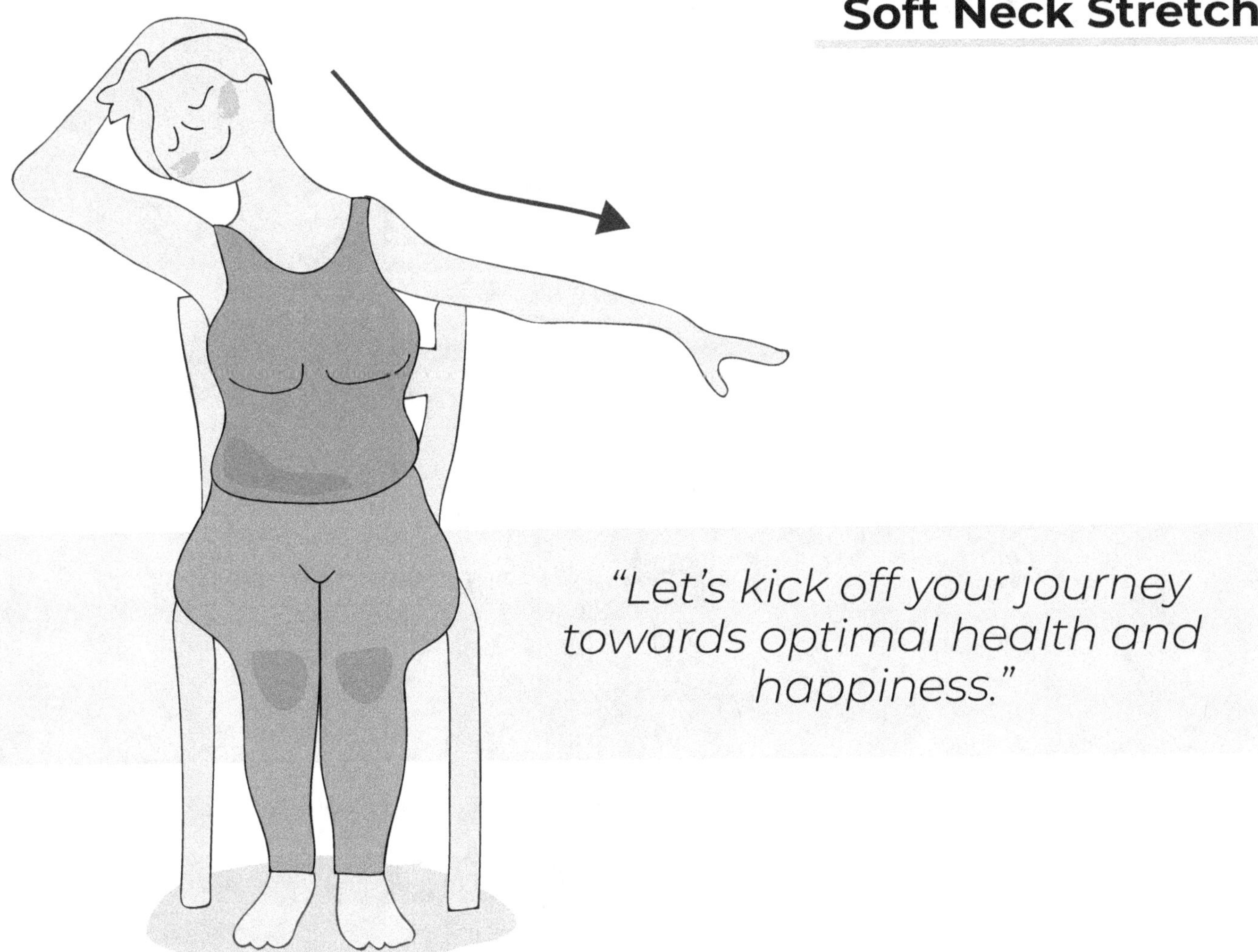

◈ Exhaling, gently place your hand on your temple and lower your right ear towards your right shoulder, keeping your opposite arm horizontal.

◈ You will experience a stretch along your neck's left side.

◈ Hold the stretch while taking a few long breaths.

◈ Inhale and lift your head to bring it back to the center.

◈ Repeat the stretch on each side for several times, moving with your breath and taking your time to stretch slowly.

Shoulder Circles

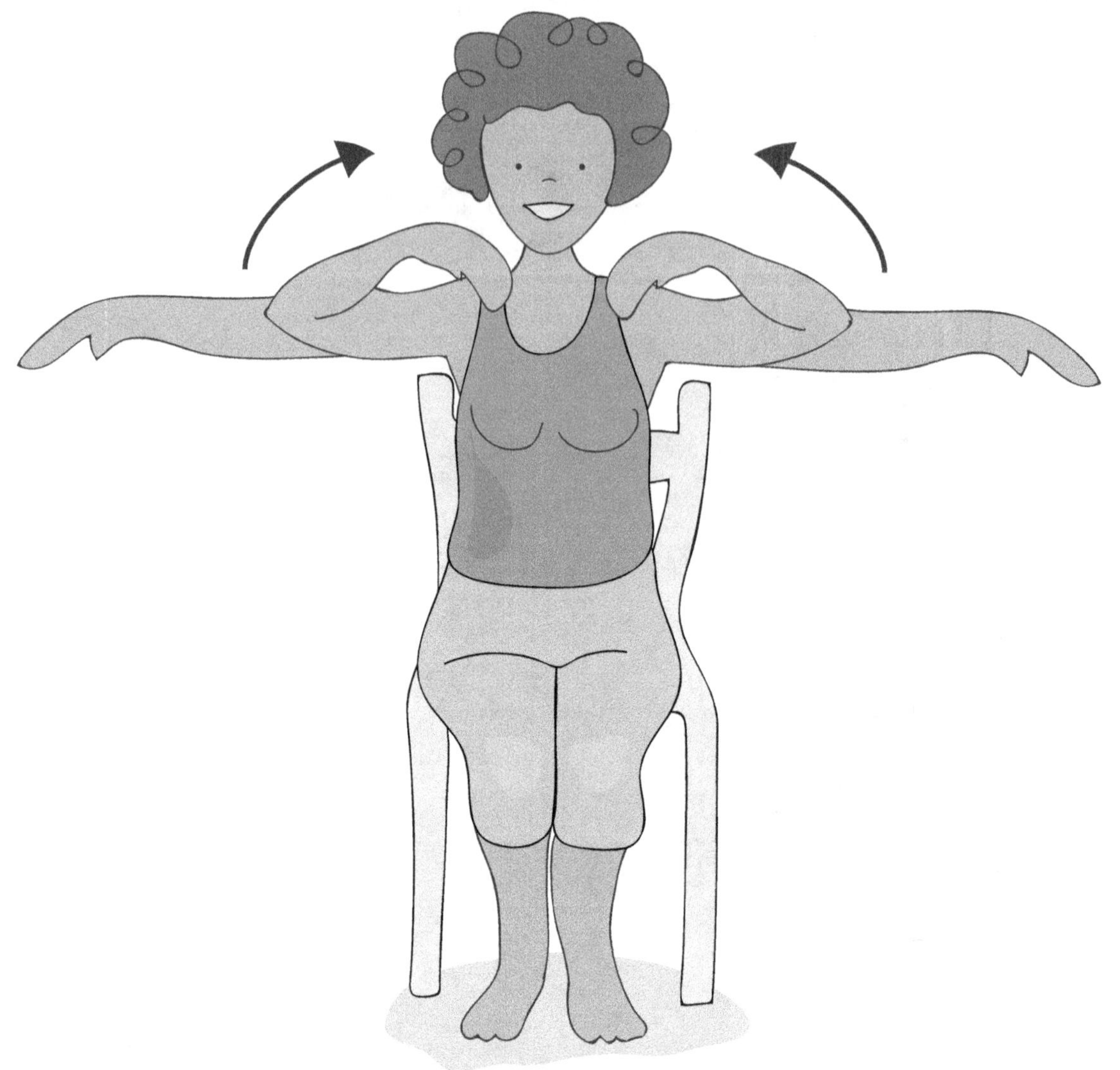

◈ Inhale and place your arms horizontally.

◈ Exhale and bend your arms until they touch your shoulders.

◈ For a little while, maintain the posture while breathing.

◈ Repeat the exercise being careful to maintain a straight back and a relaxed neck.

◈ To enhance balance, you can perform the exercise whit your eyes closed.

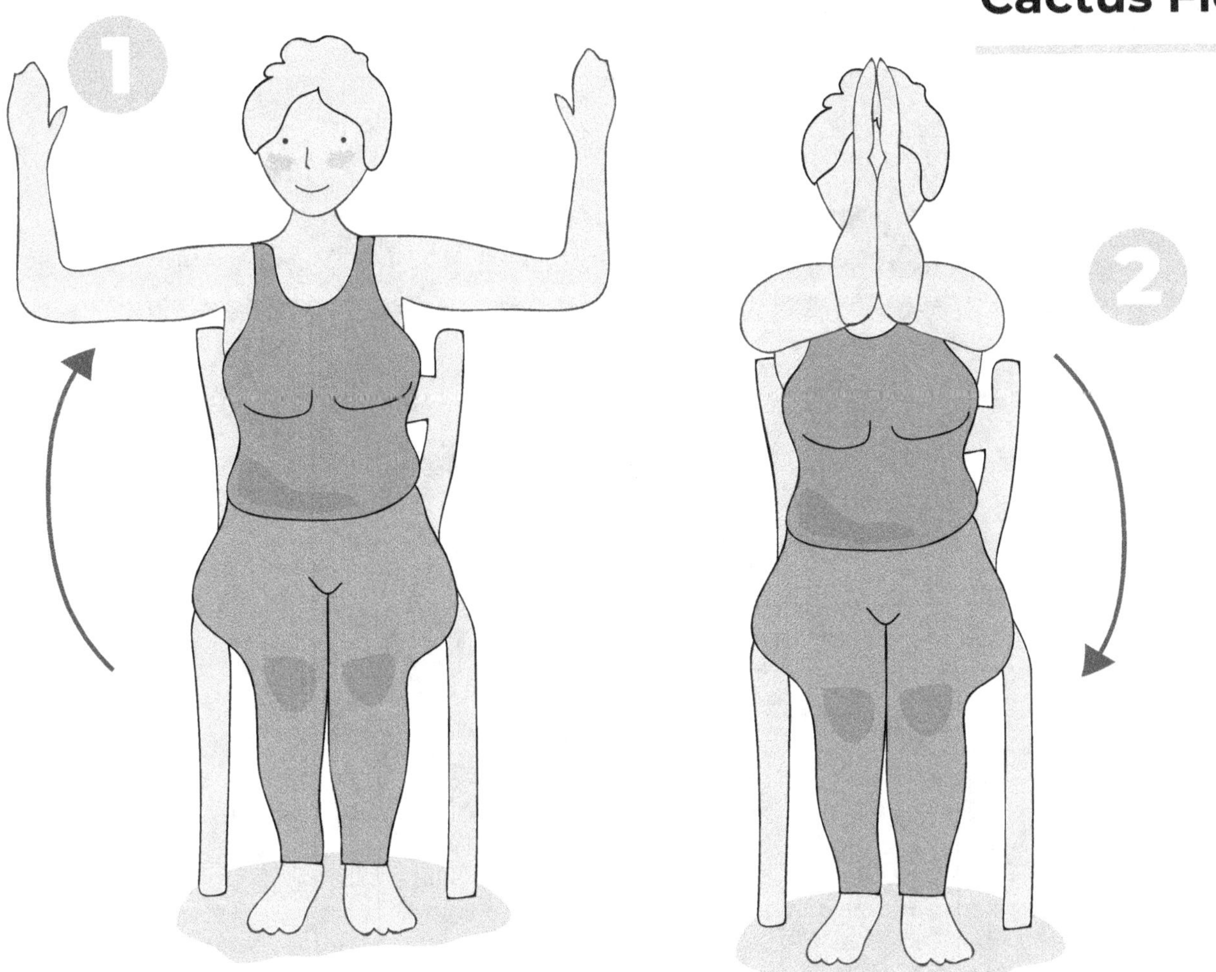

◈ Inhale and bring your arms horizontally, bending your elbows at a 90-degree angle so that your fingertips point towards the ceiling (cactus position).

◈ Exhale and let your elbows touch, widening your shoulder blades.

◈ Raise your arms back to the cactus position, opening your chest and taking a deep breath.

◈ Repeat this movement, coordinating your breath with the movements of your arms.

◈ You can perform this several times.

◈ Concentrate on the sensations in your shoulders and chest.

This is a gentle way to open your upper body and release tension.

Urdhva Hastasana

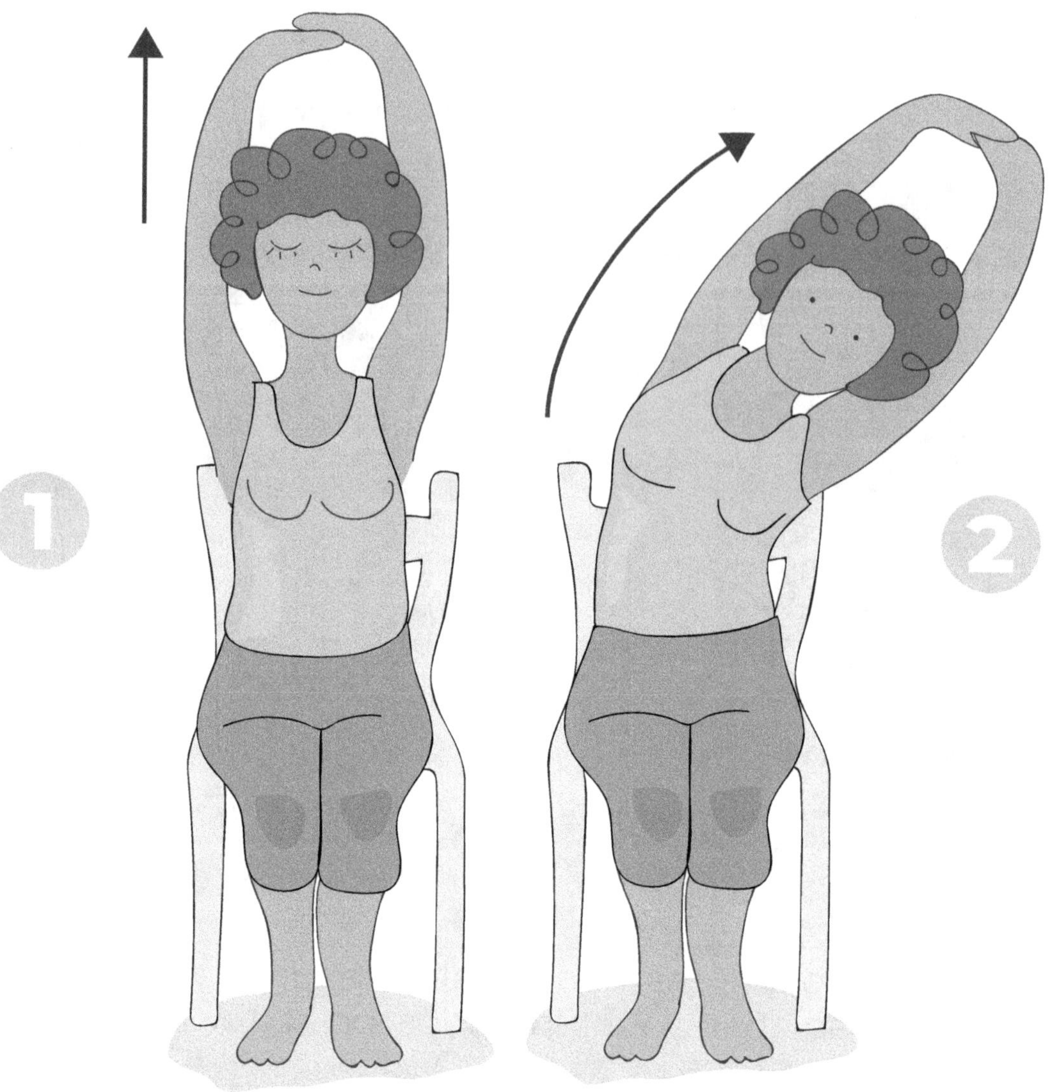

◈ Inhale and stretch your arms upwards while keeping your shoulders relaxed.

◈ While inhaling, stretch your arms even further, feeling a slight elongation of your shoulders and upper back.

◈ Hold the stretch for a few breaths.

◈ Exhale and bring your arms to one side.

◈ Repeat the exercise several times, moving with your breath and being careful not to strain your shoulders or neck.

Hands Up Pose

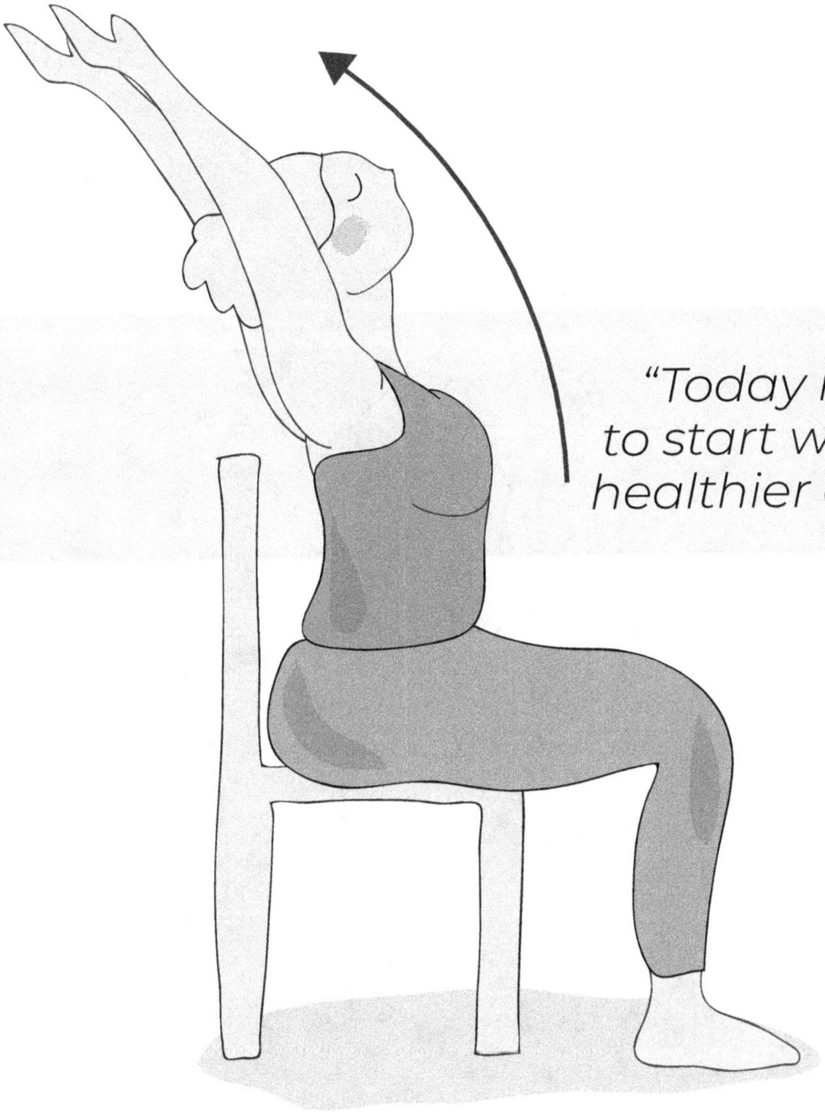

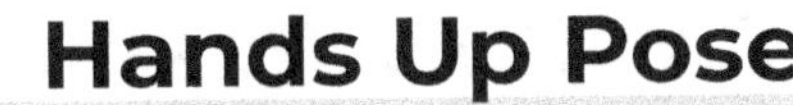

"Today is the perfect day to start working towards a healthier and happier you."

- Start in a seated position with your back straight and your hands up.
- Inhale deeply, bringing your arms behind your ears and your chin slightly upwards.
- Maintain this posture for a few breaths while relaxing your back and stomach muscles.
- Release and repeat the exercise, while staying in tune with your breathing.

When performed with eyes closed, this position can greatly relieve mental and emotional stress, enhancing your general well-being.

Cat Cow Pose

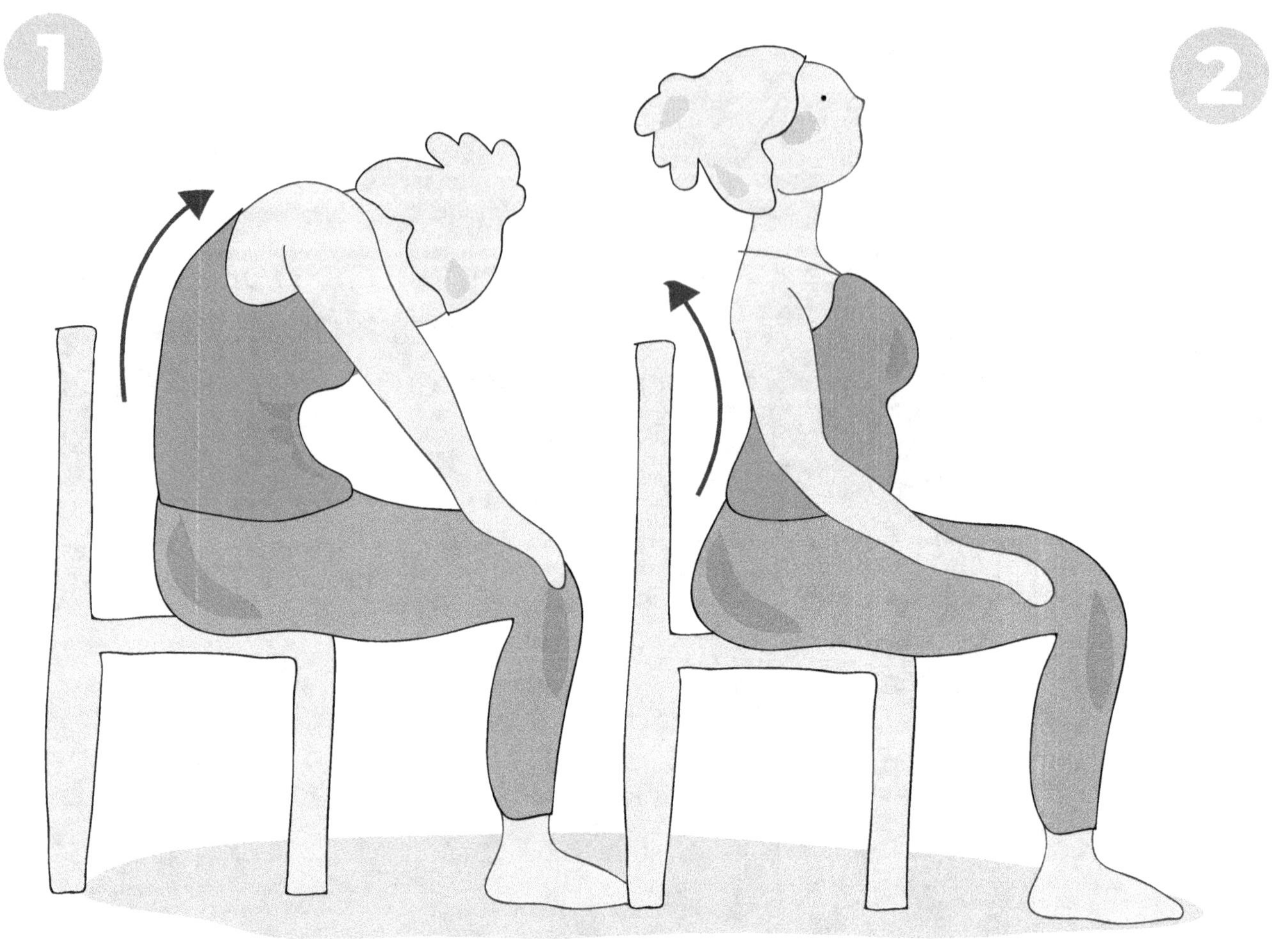

◈ As you exhale, arch your spine and gently bring your chin to your chest, pulling your shoulder blades away (cat pose).

◈ Inhaling, arch your spine and lift your chest forward, bringing your shoulder blades together (cow position).

◈ Continue alternating between these two positions with each inhalation and exhalation, concentrating on your breath's flow.

◈ Repeat for a few breaths, then return to a natural sitting position.

The Cat-Cow position is a good way to stretch and mobilize your spine, improve your posture, and relieve tension in your back and neck.

- Inhale deeply and raise your left arm towards the ceiling, lengthening your spine and stretching your left side.

- Gently lean your torso to the right, exhaling and keeping your left arm extended overhead.

- Take a few deep breaths as you hold the stretch, feeling the lengthening sensation along your left side.

- Inhale and lift your torso back to the center, lowering your left arm to your side.

- Repeat the stretch on the other side.

This pose helps to stretch and lengthen the muscles along the sides of your body, promoting improved flexibility and posture.

It can also help to relieve tension in your shoulders and back.

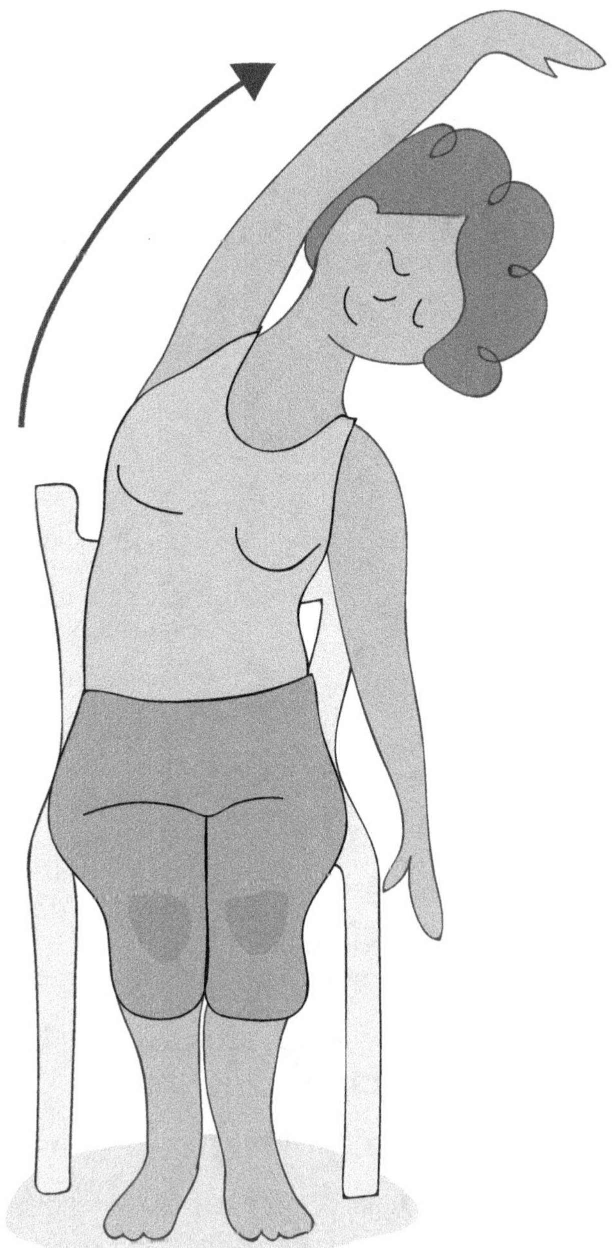

Torso Circles

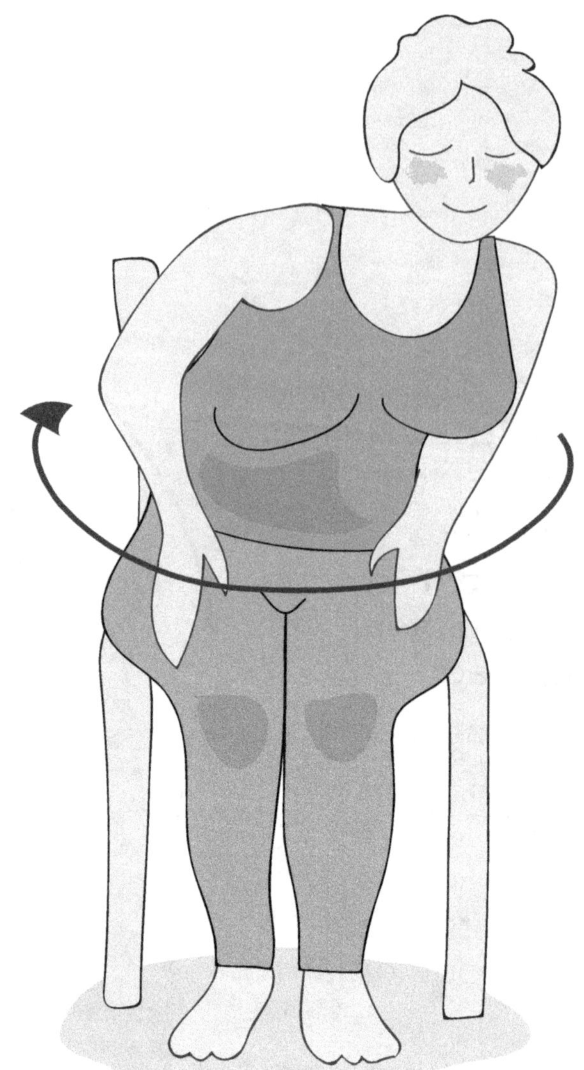

◈ Start by placing your hands on your thighs and sitting up straight in a chair with your feet firmly planted on the ground.

◈ Inhale deeply and, as you exhale, begin to rotate your upper body, guiding it with your chest and letting your head and neck follow.

◈ Repeat the circular motion several times in both directions.

◈ Pay attention to your breathing and the movement of your spine.

◈ Slowly return to the natural sitting position with your hands on your thighs.

◈ This exercise can help you increase freedom of movement, your balance, and reduce back stiffness and tension.

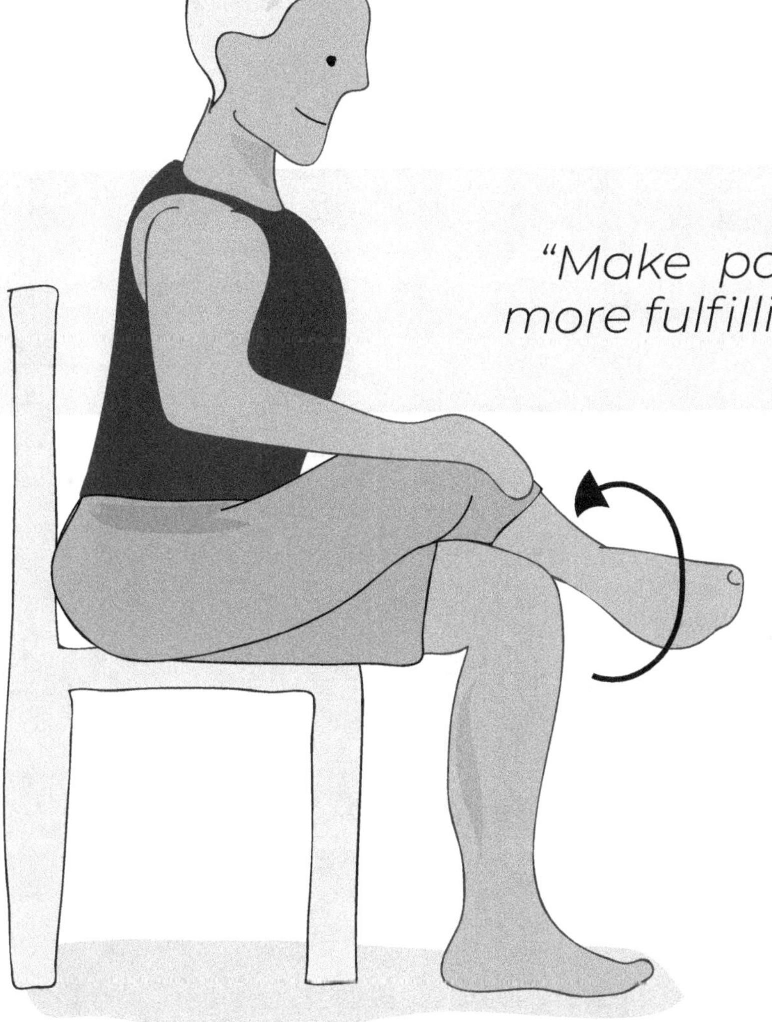

◈ Lift your foot and place your ankle on your knee.

◈ Move your ankle gently and slowly in a circle, first in one direction and then the other.

◈ Keep your torso relaxed and your posture upright.

◈ Repeat with the other side.

◈ Important: you must listen to your body and only move within a comfortable range of motion.

Flexing Foot

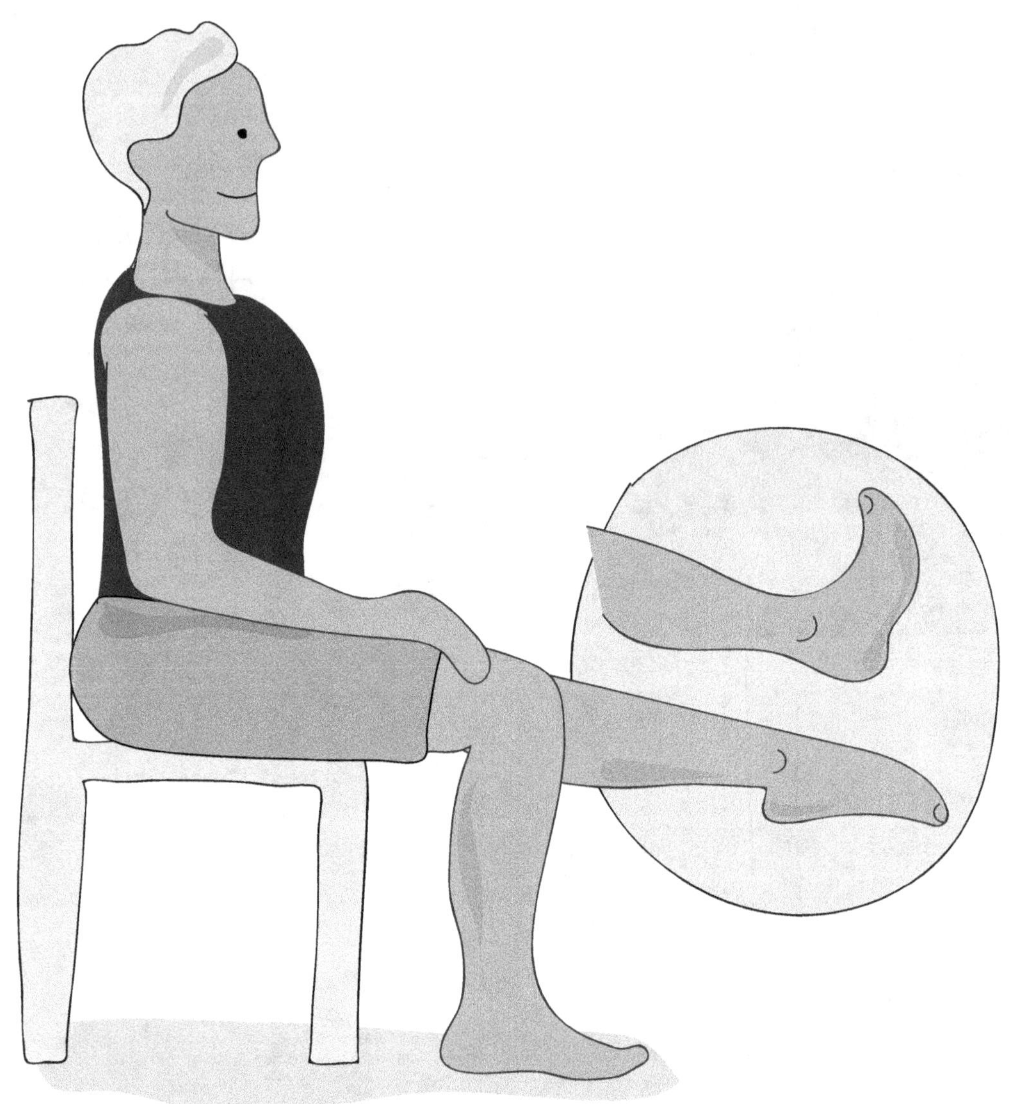

- ◈ Extend your leg straight out in front of you.
- ◈ Gently move your foot up and down, concentrating on stretching your calf and foot muscles.
- ◈ Lower your right foot to the ground and repeat the same process with your left foot.
- ◈ Perform this exercise with both feet.

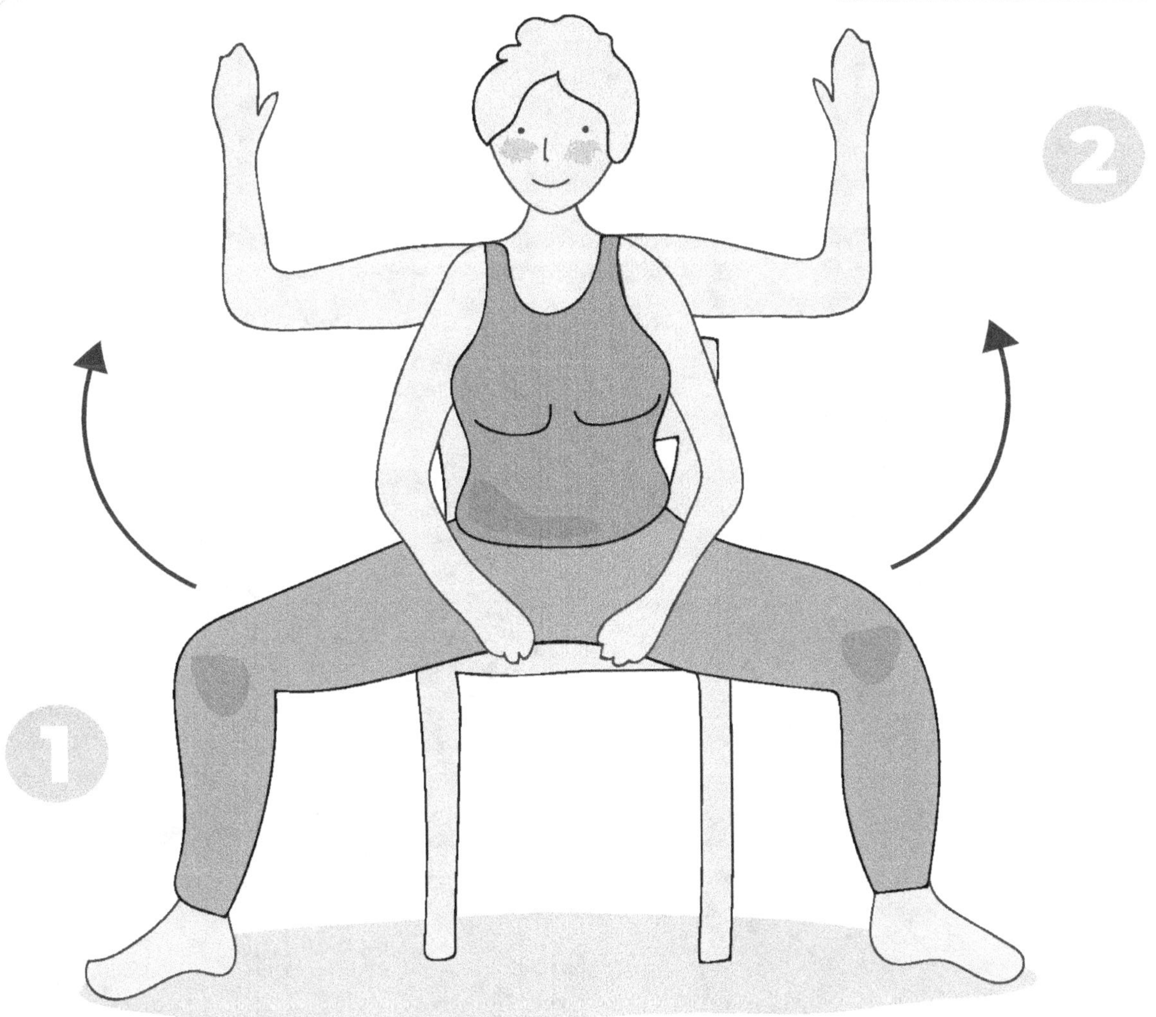

◈ Place your hands on your thighs, keep your back straight, and engage your leg muscles.

◈ Separate your thighs as wide as possible, keeping your feet and knees pointing outwards.

◈ Take a few deep breaths and hold the pose while feeling the stretch in your inner thighs and hips.

◈ Inhale while raising your arms to shoulder height, bend your elbows 90 degrees, place your palms up, and spread your fingers widely.

◈ Repeat several times.

Goddess Pose Rotated

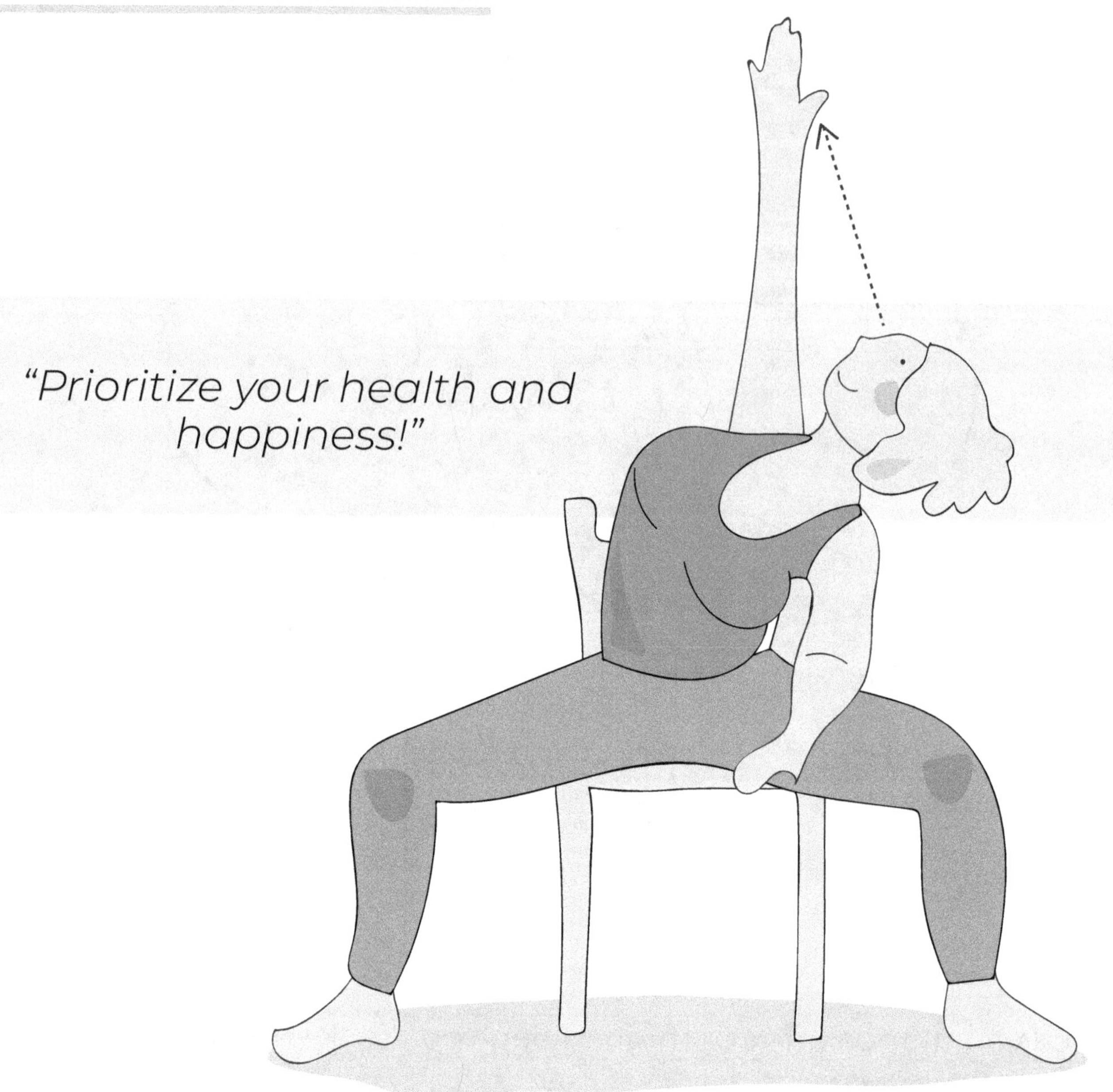

◈ Starting from the Goddess Pose, rest your arm on your thigh, and exhale.

◈ Inhale, rotate your torso, and raise your arm up high.

◈ Gently rotate your head and look at your fingertips.

◈ For a few breaths, hold this posture, and then exhale.

◈ Repeat with the other side.

Half Forward Fold Pose

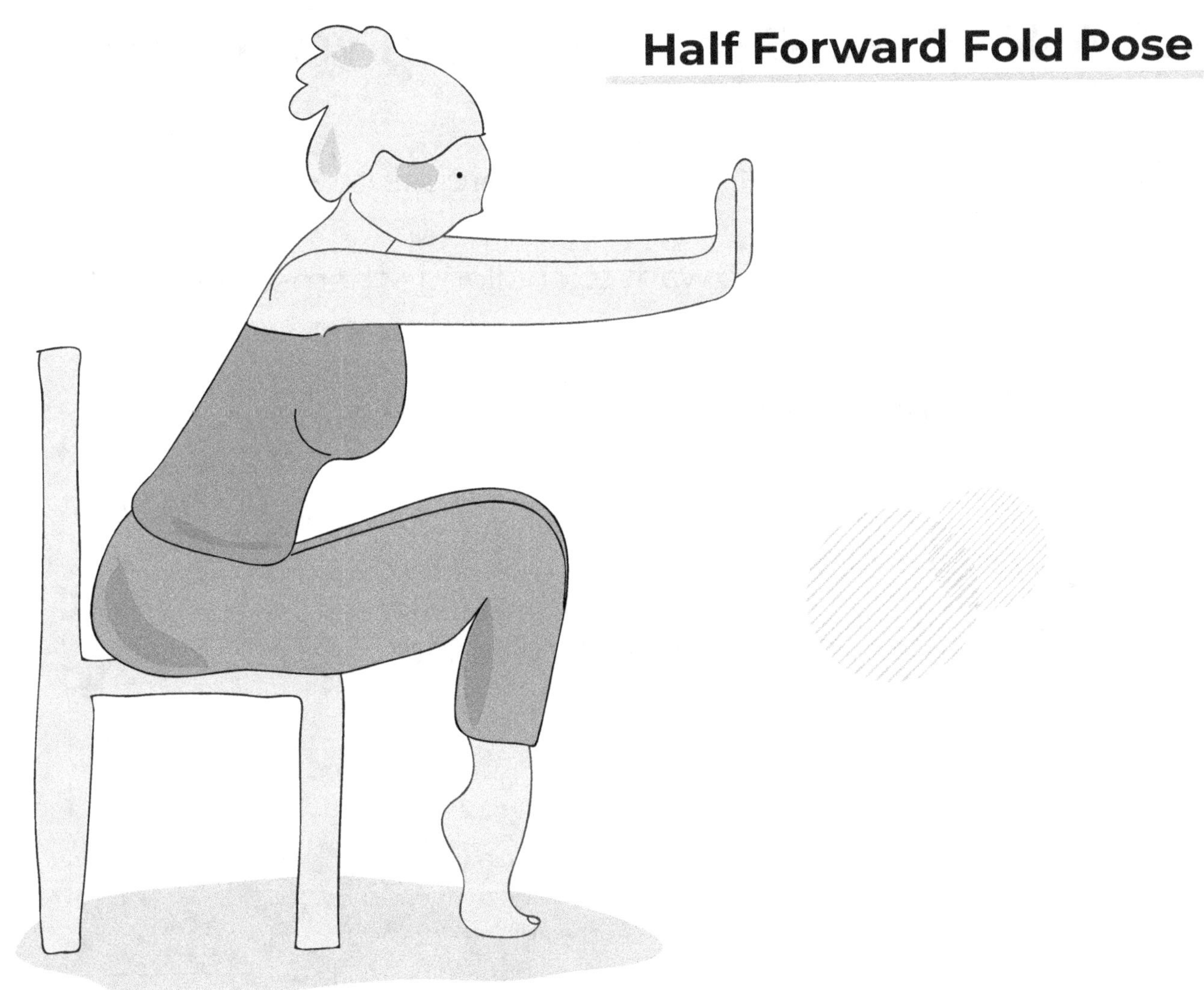

◈ Stretch out your arms in front of you with your fingers pointing upwards, and inhale.

◈ Exhaling, slowly bend your hips forward, keeping your back flat.

◈ Lift your heels off the floor and keep your neck parallel to your back with your head relaxed.

◈ Hold for a few breaths while feeling the stretch in your back and behind your thighs.

◈ Finally, inhale and slowly raise your torso to a sitting position.

This exercise helps to increase flexibility, reduce back stress, and enhance posture.

ADVANCED POSES 'DEEPENING YOUR PRACTICE'

This pose includes advanced-level exercises to stretch and tone your deep muscles.

It is suitable for those who want to challenge themselves further in their yoga practice.

Pose Blanket Roll Back

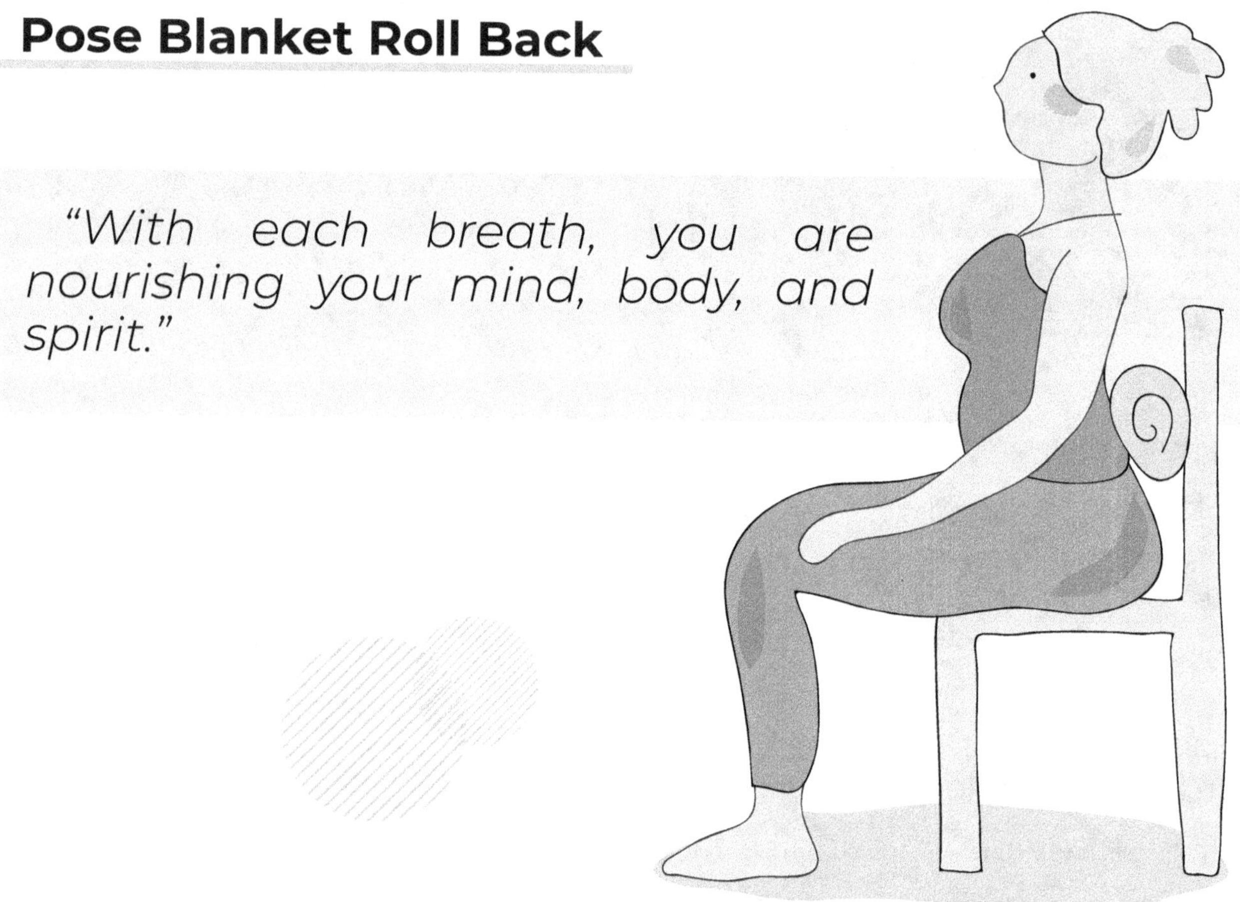

"With each breath, you are nourishing your mind, body, and spirit."

◈ Sit on a chair with a pillow or a folded blanket behind your back.

Take a few deep breaths, holding this position.

The benefits of this exercise include reduced tension and pain in your lower back, stress relief, and increased awareness of your breath and body.

Remember to adjust your posture if necessary and to listen to your body.

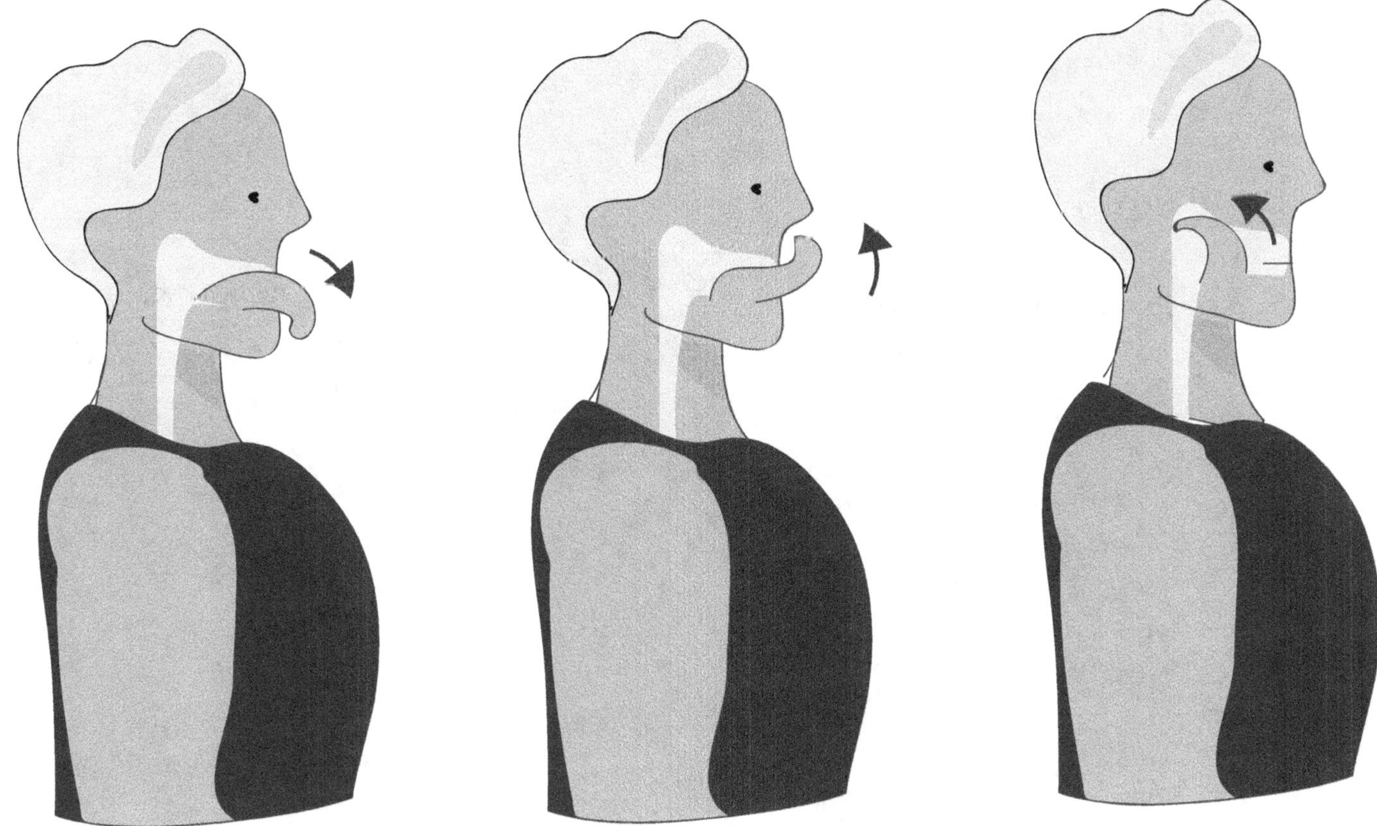

◈ Exhale and extend your tongue out of your mouth, bringing the tip downwards.

◈ Take a few deep breaths, then while exhaling, touch the tip of your nose with your tongue.

◈ Then, with your mouth shut, briefly massage the palate with your tongue.

◈ After a few breaths, revert to your natural position.

This exercise is useful for relaxing your face and jaw muscles and relieving your mouth.

Eagle Arms Pose

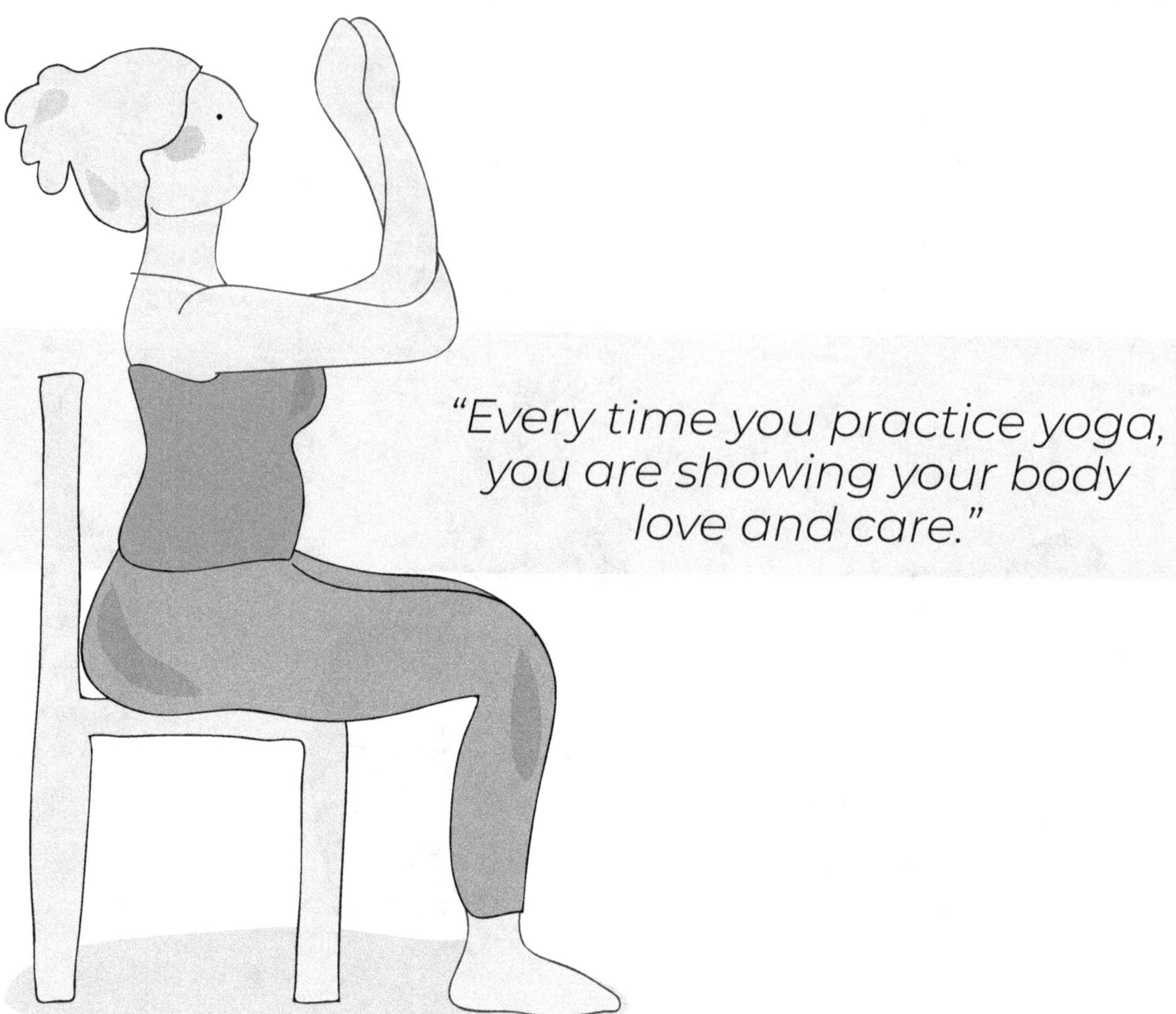

◈ Raise your arms in front of you to your shoulder height and cross your right arm over your left arm at the elbows, palms down.

◈ Bend your arms and bring the back of your hands to touch, or as close as possible.

◈ If it feels comfortable, lift your elbows slightly and press the back of your hands together firmly.

◈ Hold this position while taking several deep breaths, then release and switch arms.

This position helps to stretch your shoulders and upper back and can also improve concentration and balance.

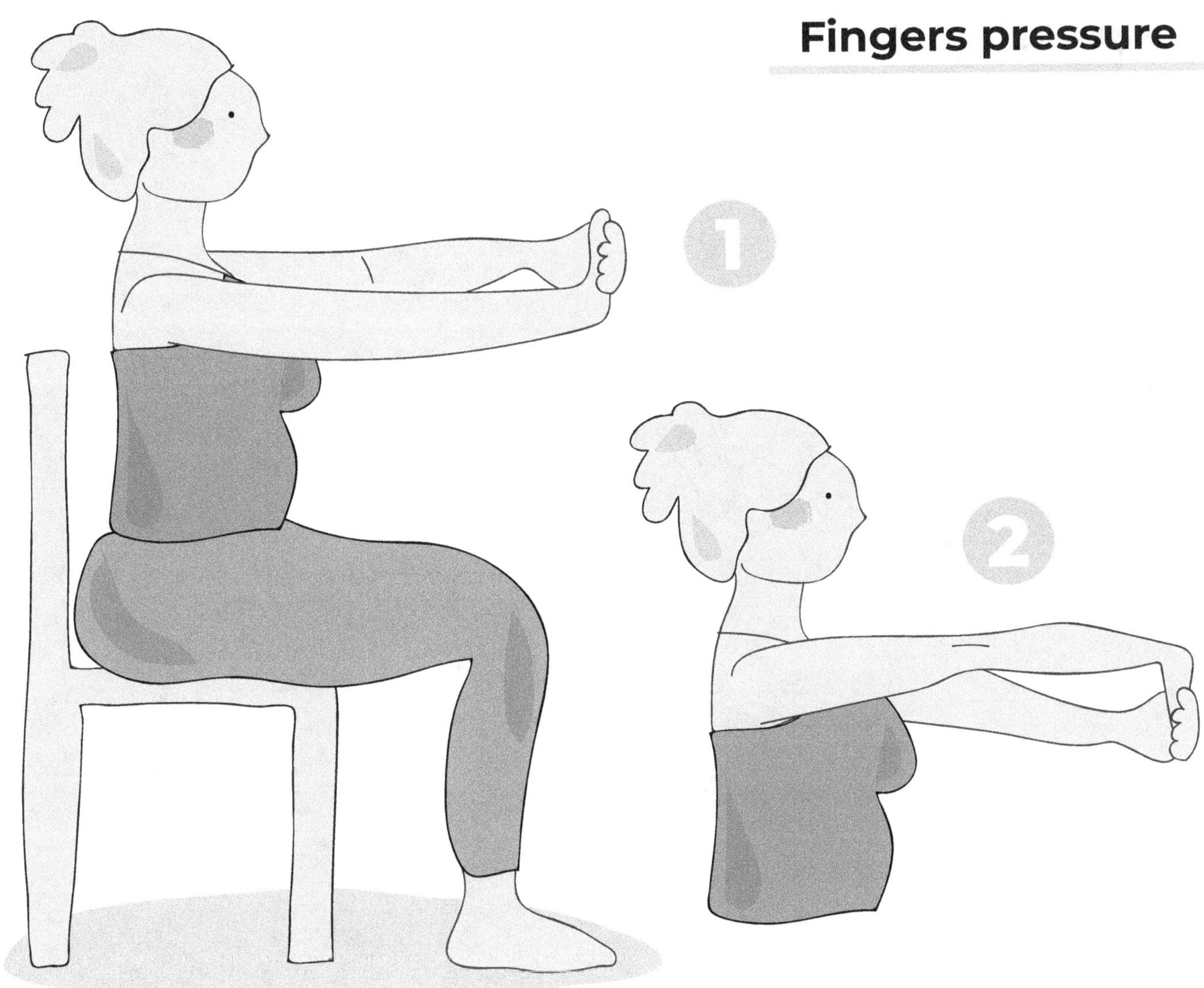

◈ Stretch out one arm forward with your fingers pointing upwards.

◈ With your other hand, grasp your fingers and while exhaling, stretch your palm towards you.

◈ Hold this position for a few breaths.

◈ Now turn your fingers downwards and while exhaling, stretch your fingers towards you.

◈ For a few breaths, maintain this posture.

◈ Repeat with the other arm.

This exercise helps relieve the tension in your hands, wrists, and arms.

Namaskar Mudra

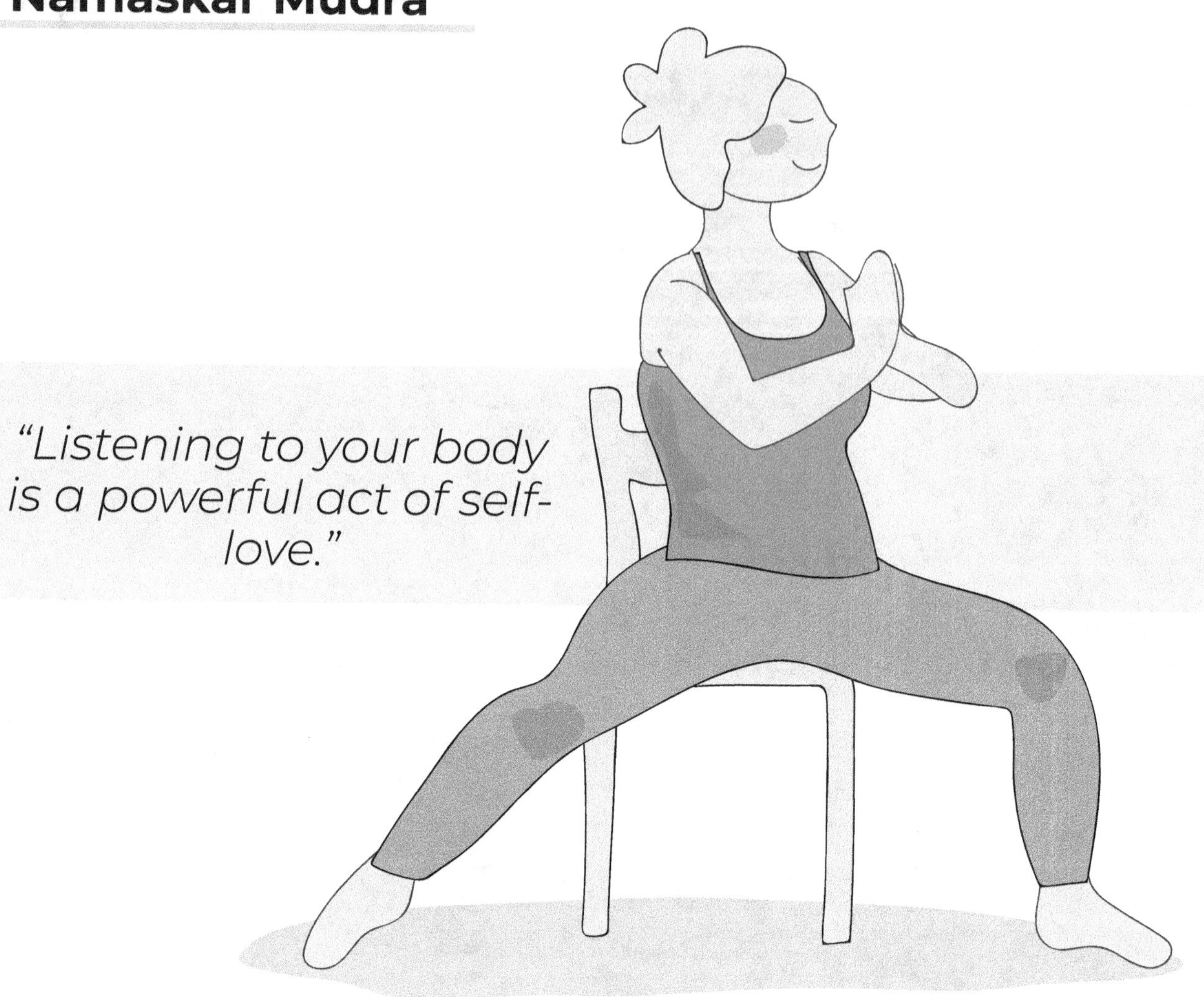

◈ Inhale and extend your leg outwards.

◈ Exhaling, slowly start to turn your torso carefully, coordinating the movement with your breath.

◈ Bring your hands together in prayer and hold the position for a few breaths, feeling the elongation of your thighs and hips.

◈ When you are ready to release, inhale, then center yourself, sitting upright. Repeat with the opposite side.

This is a great way to release tension and energize your body, especially during long periods of sitting.

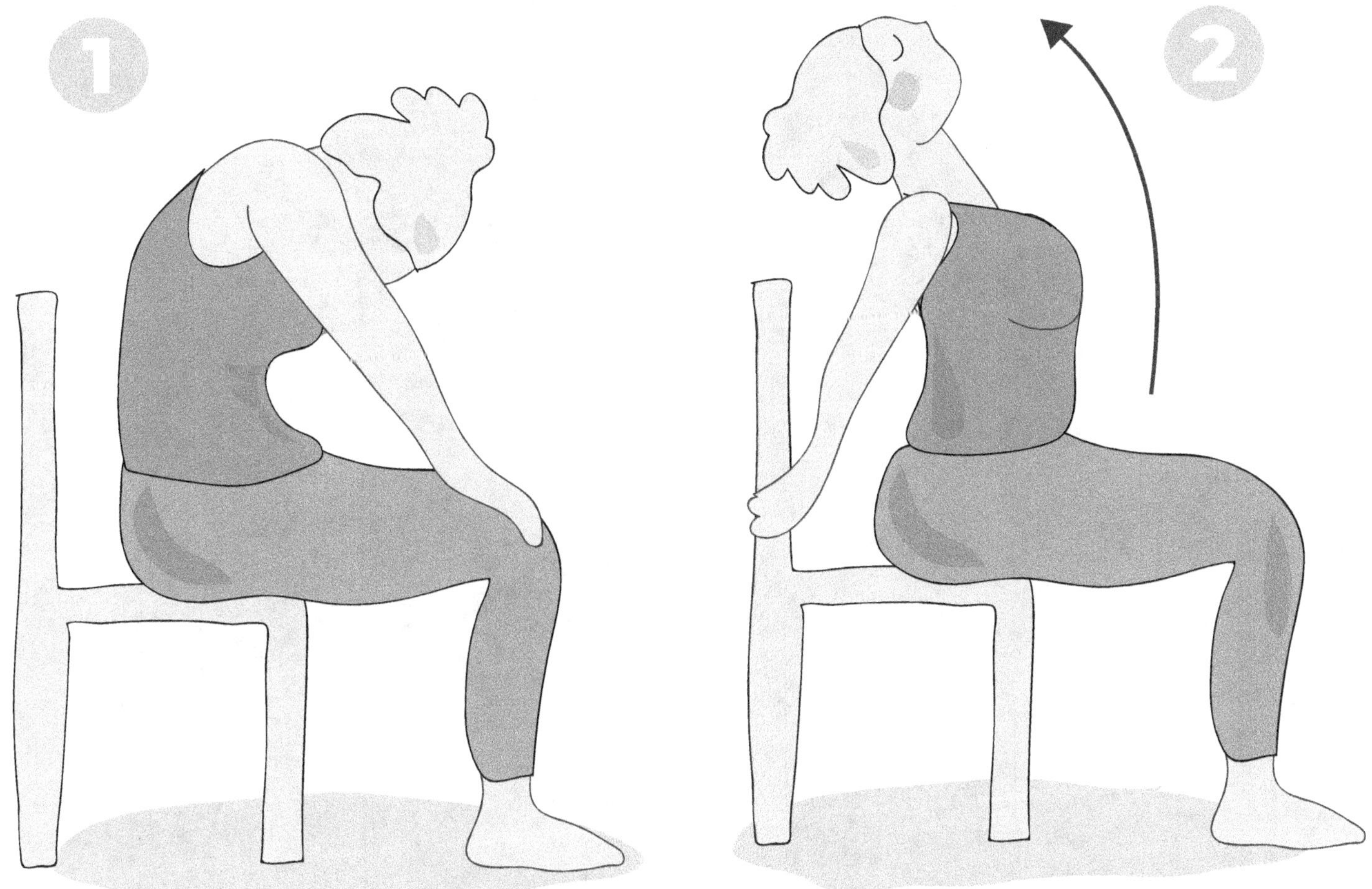

◈ Start by sitting tall on the chair with your hands resting on your thighs, and inhale.

◈ Arch your spine and bring your chin to your chest as you exhale, separating your shoulder blades (cat pose).

◈ Arch your back, take a deep breath and raise your chest forward while clenching your shoulder blades.

◈ Bring your arms towards the backrest of the chair in the half arch pose, and look up.

Hold this position for a few seconds, then slowly sit back down.

This is a good way to improve your posture, and relieve tension in your neck.

Elbow Flow Rounded Back

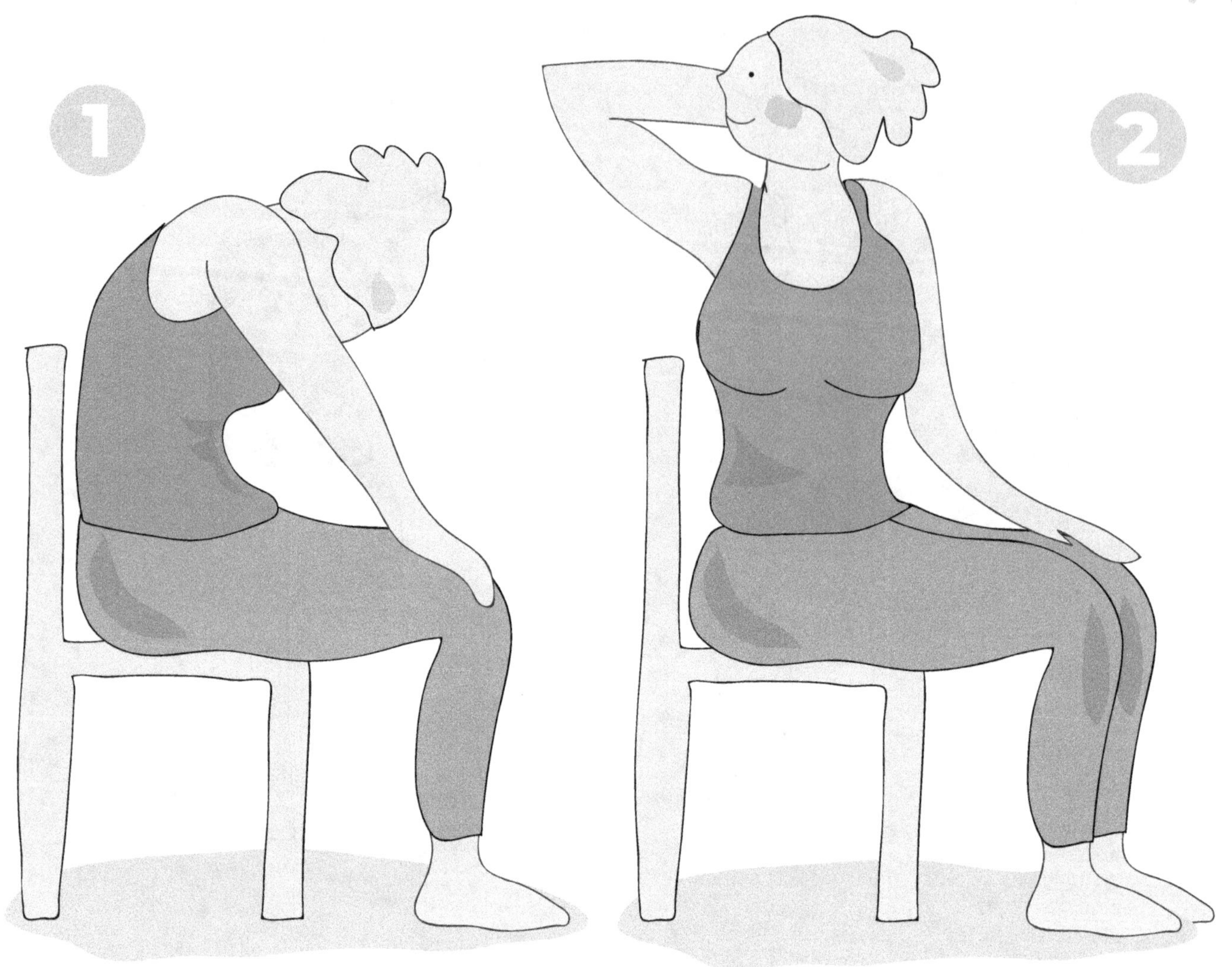

◈ Start with a rounded back and your hands on your thighs.

◈ Inhale and open your elbows, straightening your torso.

◈ Bring your gaze towards your elbows. Exhale returning to the starting position.

◈ Repeat this exercise with the other side.

◈ Alternate this movement several times, coordinating your breathing with the movement.

This position helps improve strength, balance, and flexibility, as well as stretching your back muscles.

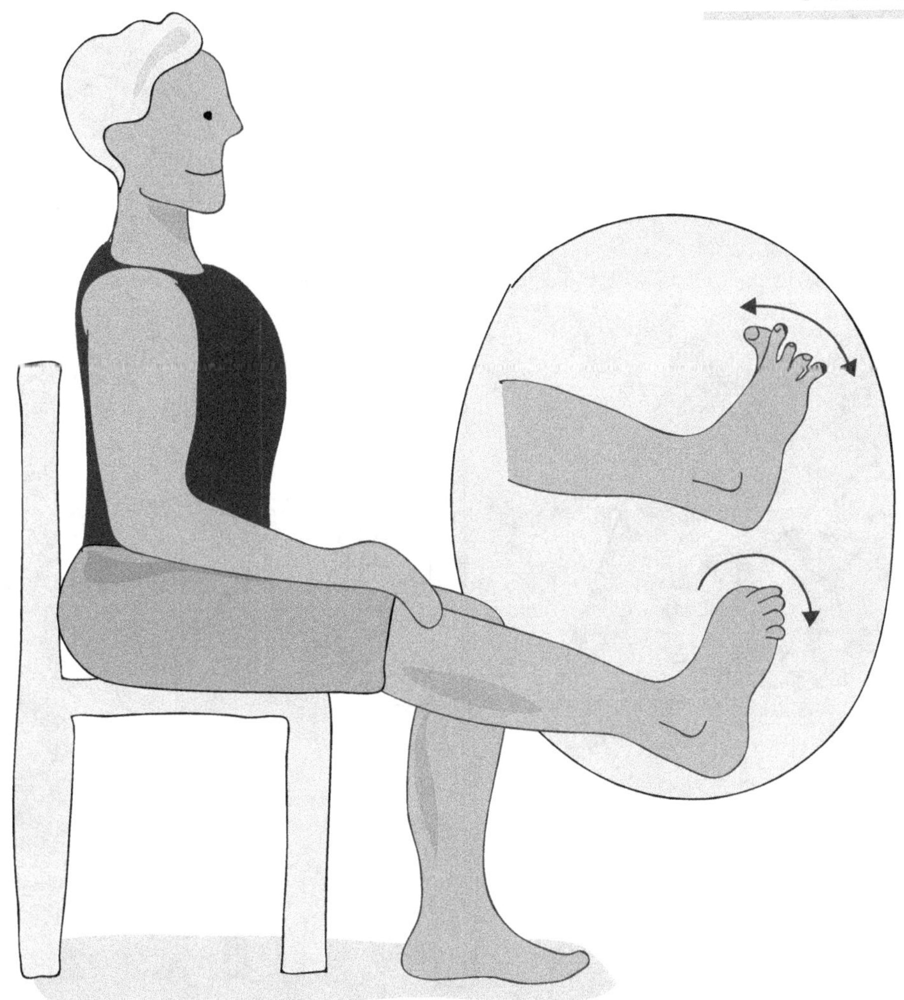

◈ Perform this toe-stretching exercise slowly.

◈ Stretch your toes upwards and hold for a few breaths.

◈ Then, bring your toes downwards and hold for a few breaths.

◈ Pay attention to the stretching of your tendons, muscles, and ligaments.

This exercise is effective for strengthening and stabilizing your ankles, improving foot health, and providing greater stability by supporting the weight of your body.

Low Lunge

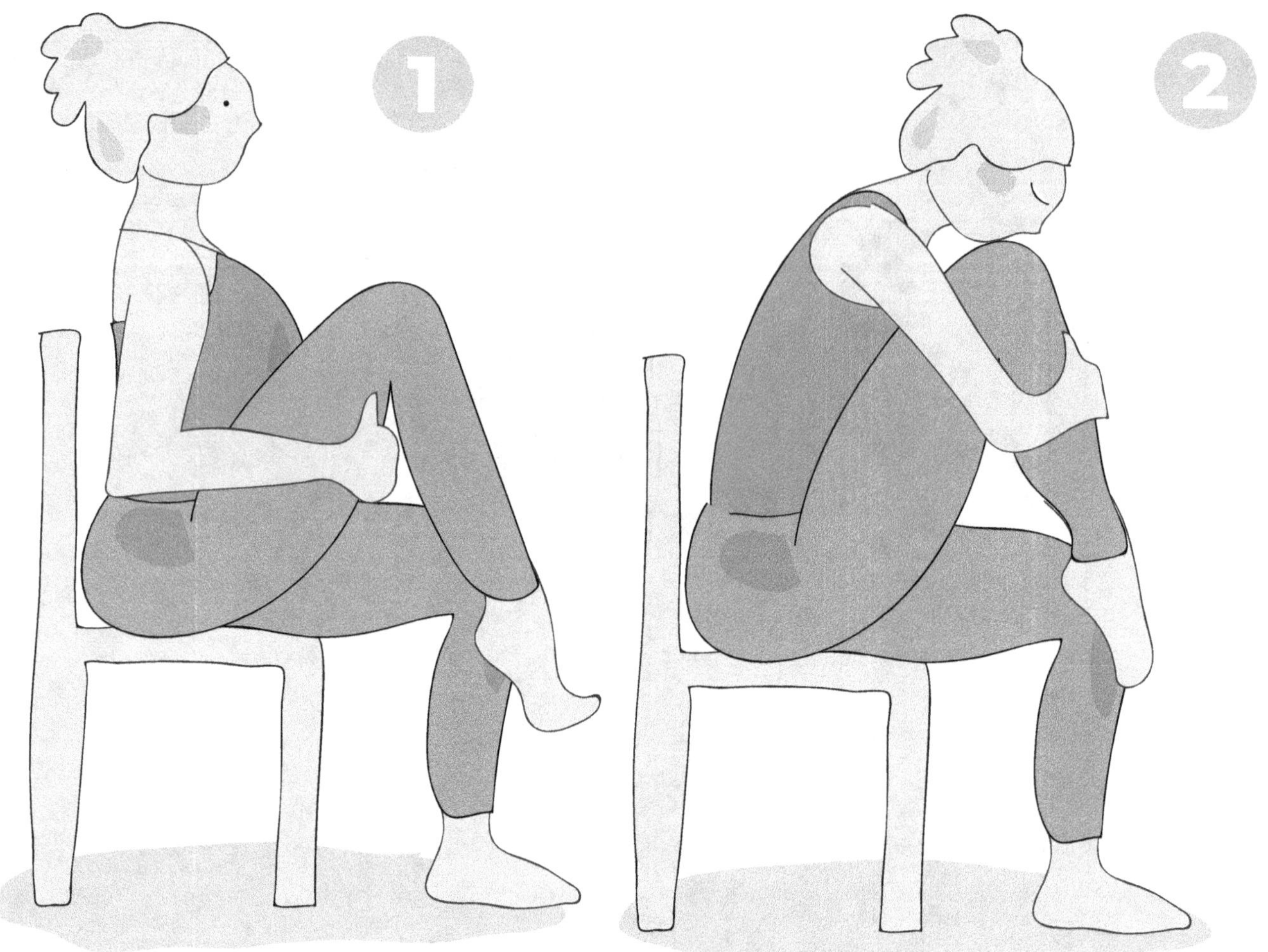

◈ Lift one foot off the ground while exhaling.

◈ Bring your thigh against your chest with the help of your hands.

◈ Breathe in and stretch your spine, staring in front of you.

◈ Exhale and rest your forehead on your knee gently, only as far as you feel comfortable.

◈ Be sure to stop before you experience any discomfort or pain.

◈ Hold this position while breathing deeply and relaxing.

◈ To return to a natural position, release your hands and gently lift your body up to a seated position.

◈ Repeat with the other leg.

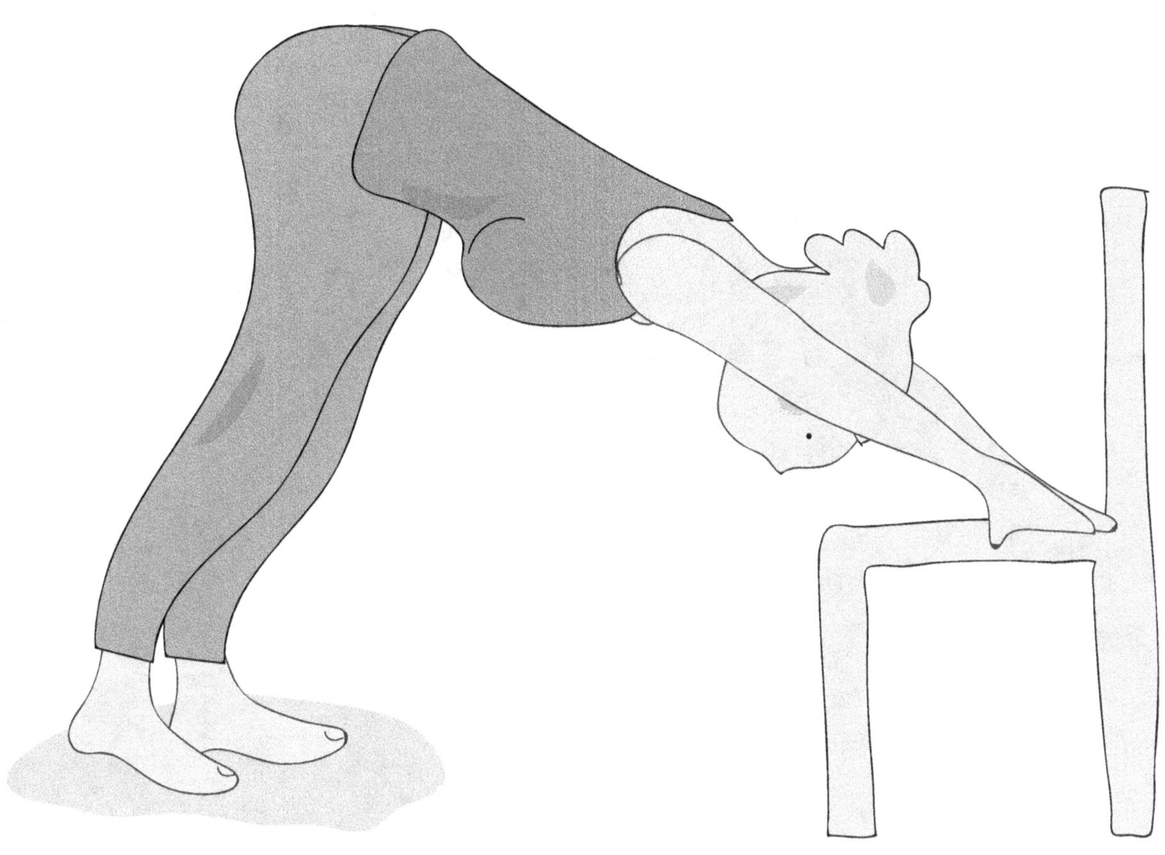

◈ Stand and place your hands on the chair with your head between your arms.

◈ Keep your legs stretched out and hold this position for a few deep breaths, feeling the stretch in your shoulders and legs.

This position can help stretch your spine, hamstrings, and shoulders. It can also improve blood circulation and help relieve stress and tension in your body.

Leaning Forward

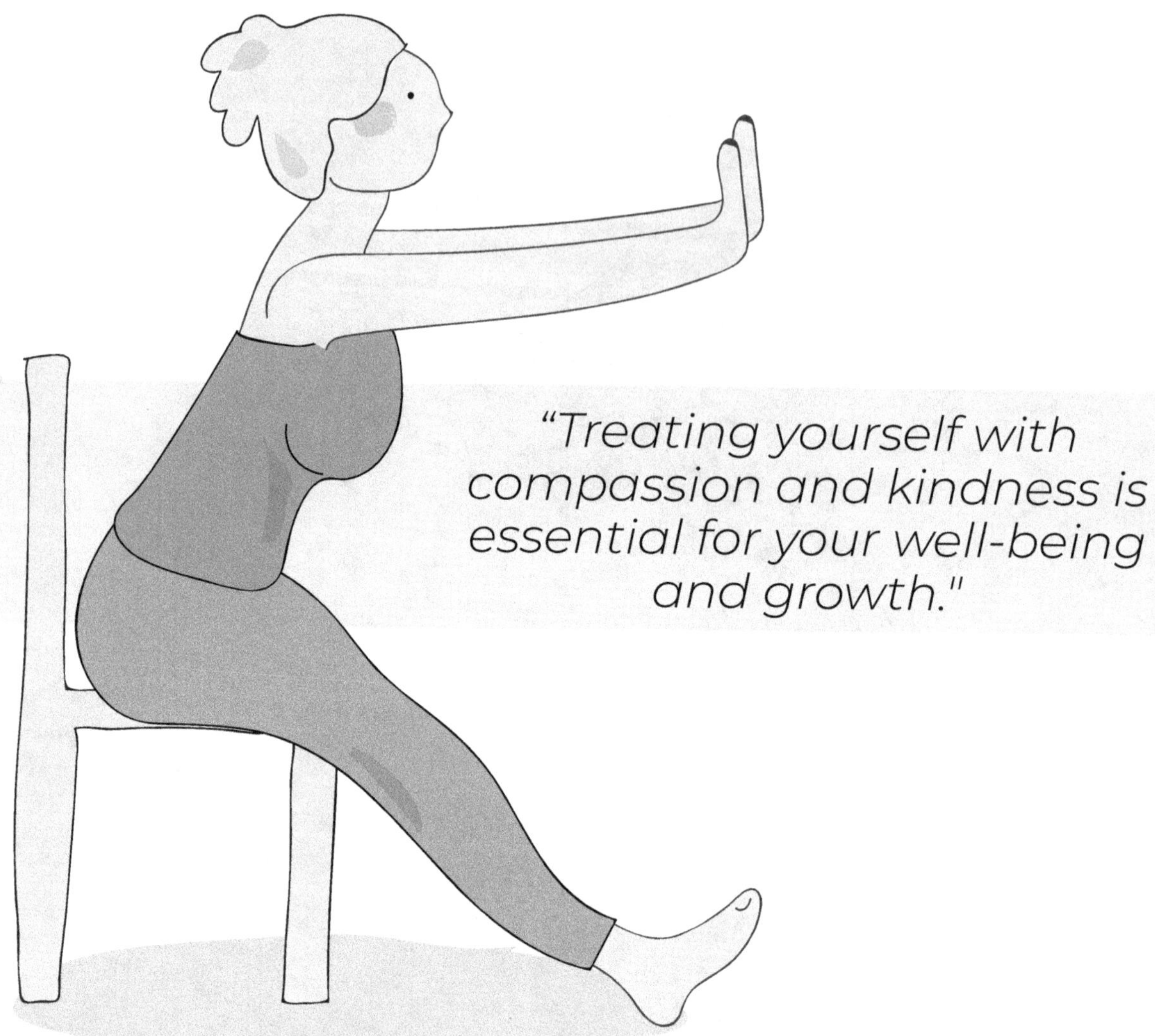

◈ Stretch out your arms in front of you with your fingers pointing upwards, as you inhale.

◈ Exhaling, slowly bend forward at your sides, keeping your back flat.

◈ Your toes should be pointing upward when you extend your legs out in front of you.

◈ Keep your neck in line with your back and relax your head.

◈ While feeling your back and thighs stretch, hold the pose for a few breaths.

◈ To release, inhale, and slowly lift your torso up to a sitting position.

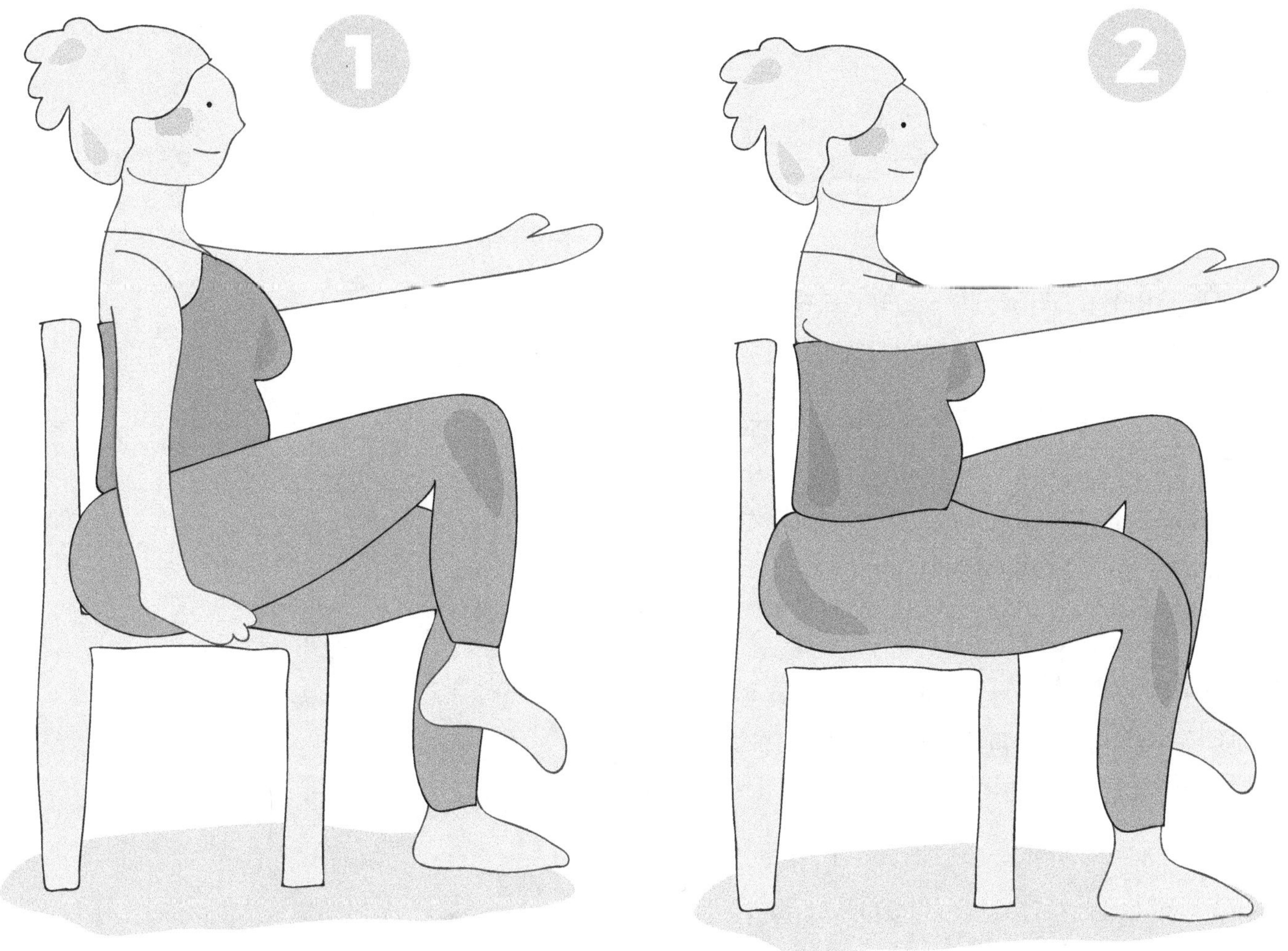

- ◈ While sitting, inhale and raise one knee and the opposite arm horizontally in front of you.

- ◈ Exhaling, return to the seated position.

- ◈ Slowly alternate the exercise with the opposite leg and arm, following your rhythmic breathing.

- ◈ Ensure that your back is straight.

- ◈ After a few repetitions, return to the seated position.

Parsva Sukhasana Garudasana

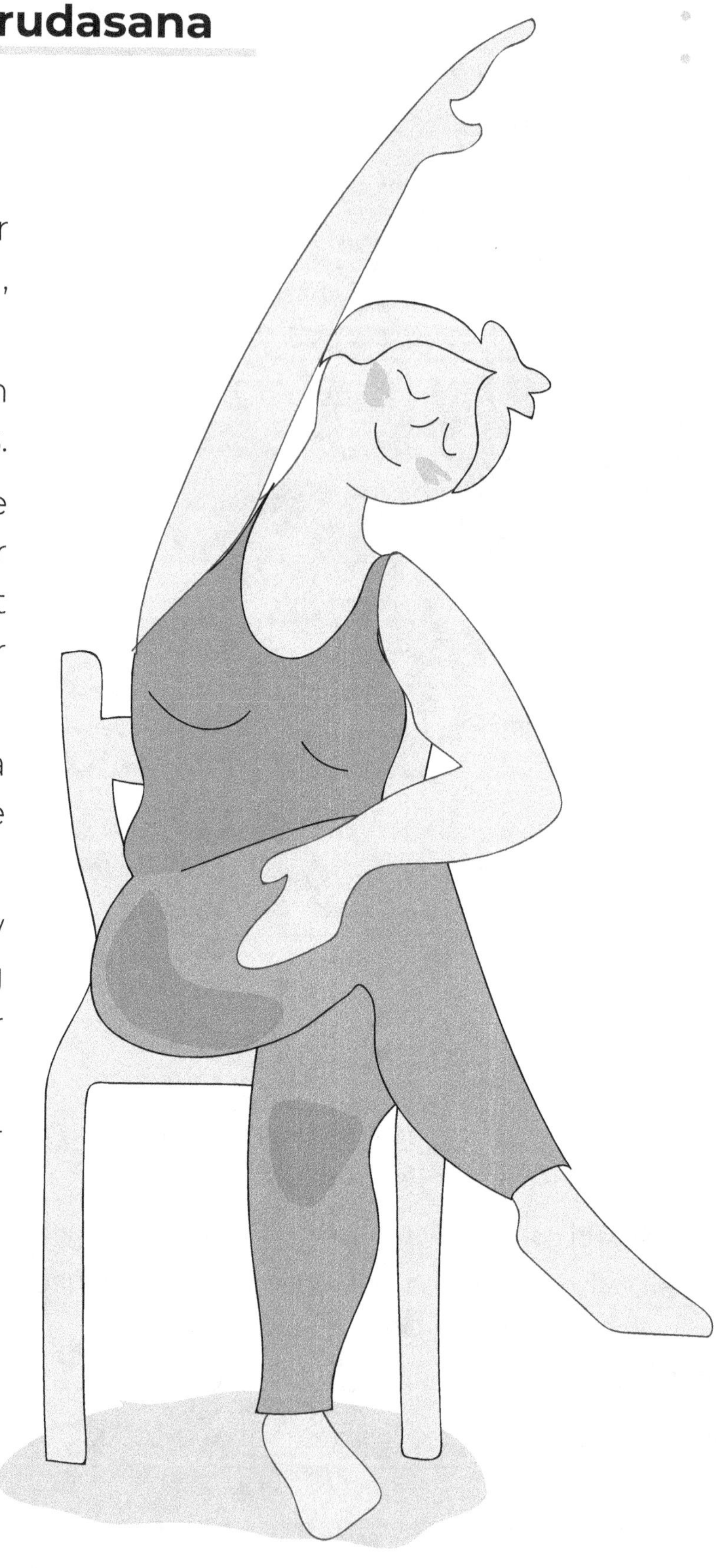

◈ Start by sitting on the chair with your legs crossed, stretching your spine.

◈ Inhaling, raise the same arm as your crossed leg upwards.

◈ If possible, deepen the stretch by placing your other hand on your bent knee and gently bring your leg towards your chest.

◈ Maintain this position for a few long deep breaths while feeling your side extend.

◈ Release and sit for a few breaths before repeating the exercise with the other side.

Always pay attention to your body and follow your instincts.

Parivrtta Utkatasana

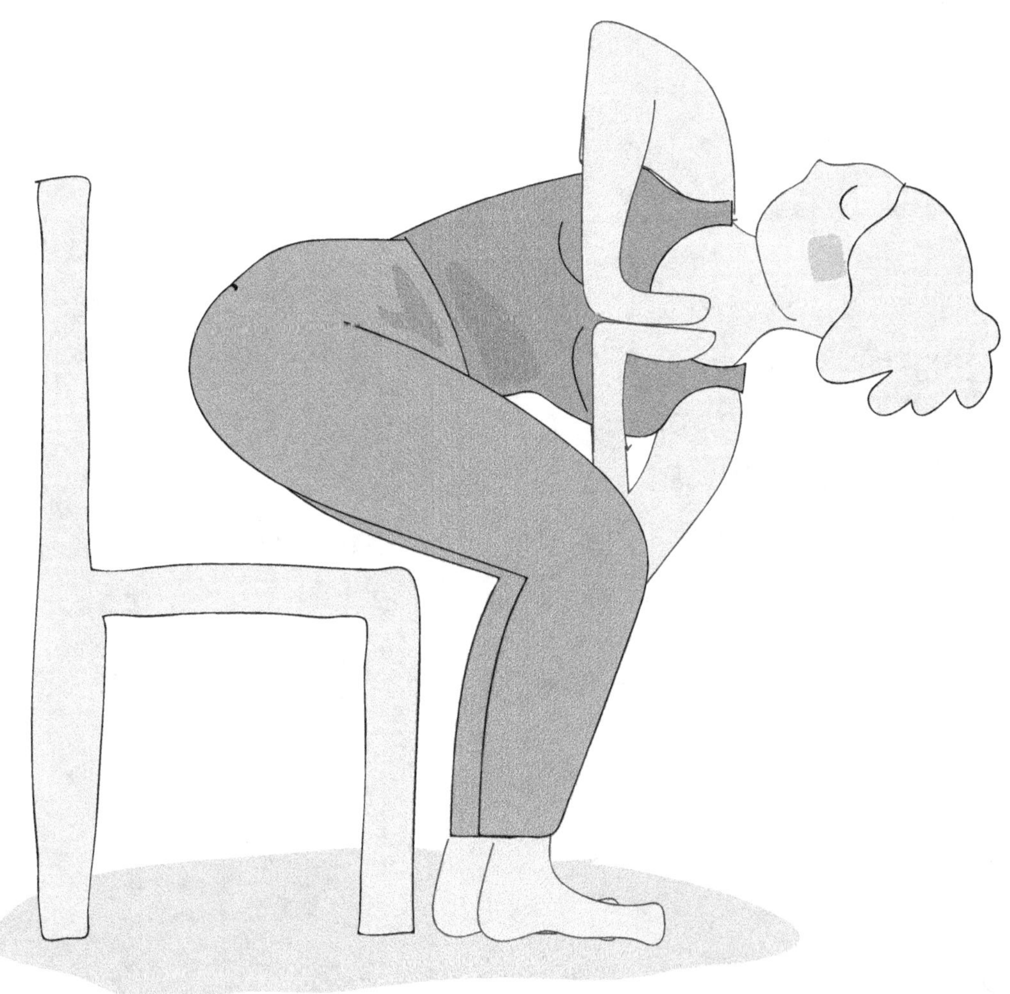

◈ Start by sitting with your back straight.

◈ Place your hands at the center of your chest, in a prayer gesture.

◈ Rotate your torso to one side, exhaling. If possible, gently stand up, with your weight on your feet firmly planted on the ground.

◈ Hold this position for a few seconds.

◈ To release, inhale and return to the center.

◈ Repeat this exercise with the other side.

Pigeon Pose Variation

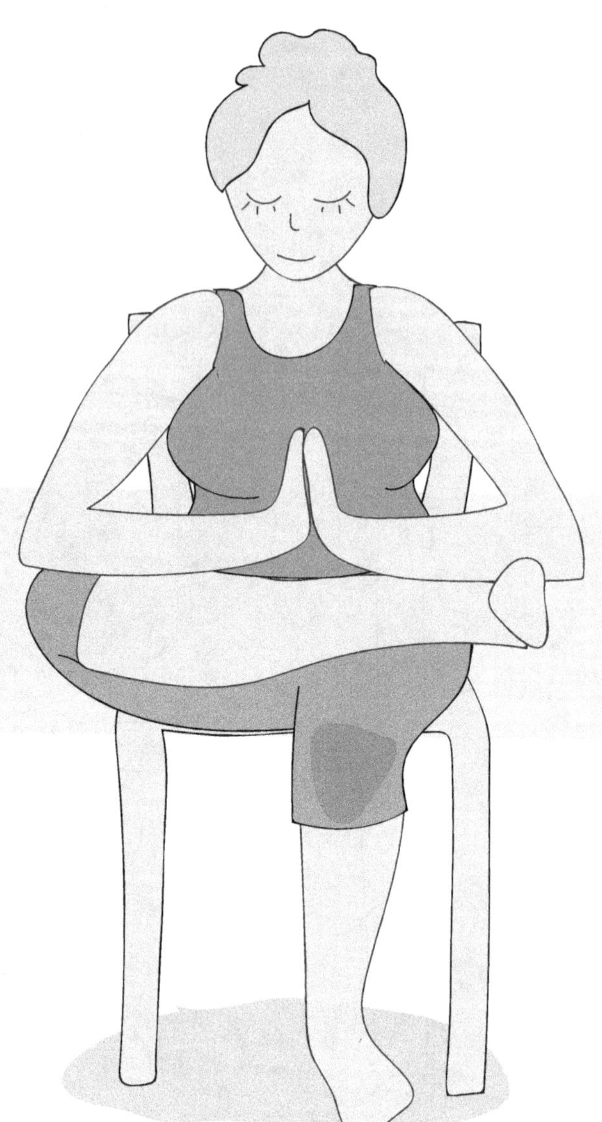

◈ Place one ankle on the opposite thigh, just above your knee.

◈ Inhale and stretch your spine, placing your hands in front of you, in prayer.

◈ Exhaling, gently bend forward, bringing your chest towards your legs.

◈ Keep your head and back in alignment.

◈ Hold this posture for a few breaths while feeling your hips stretch.

◈ Release slowly and take a few breaths.

◈ Repeat this exercise with the other side.

◈ Return to the seated position for a few breaths, listening to your body.

Pigeon Pose Palms Up

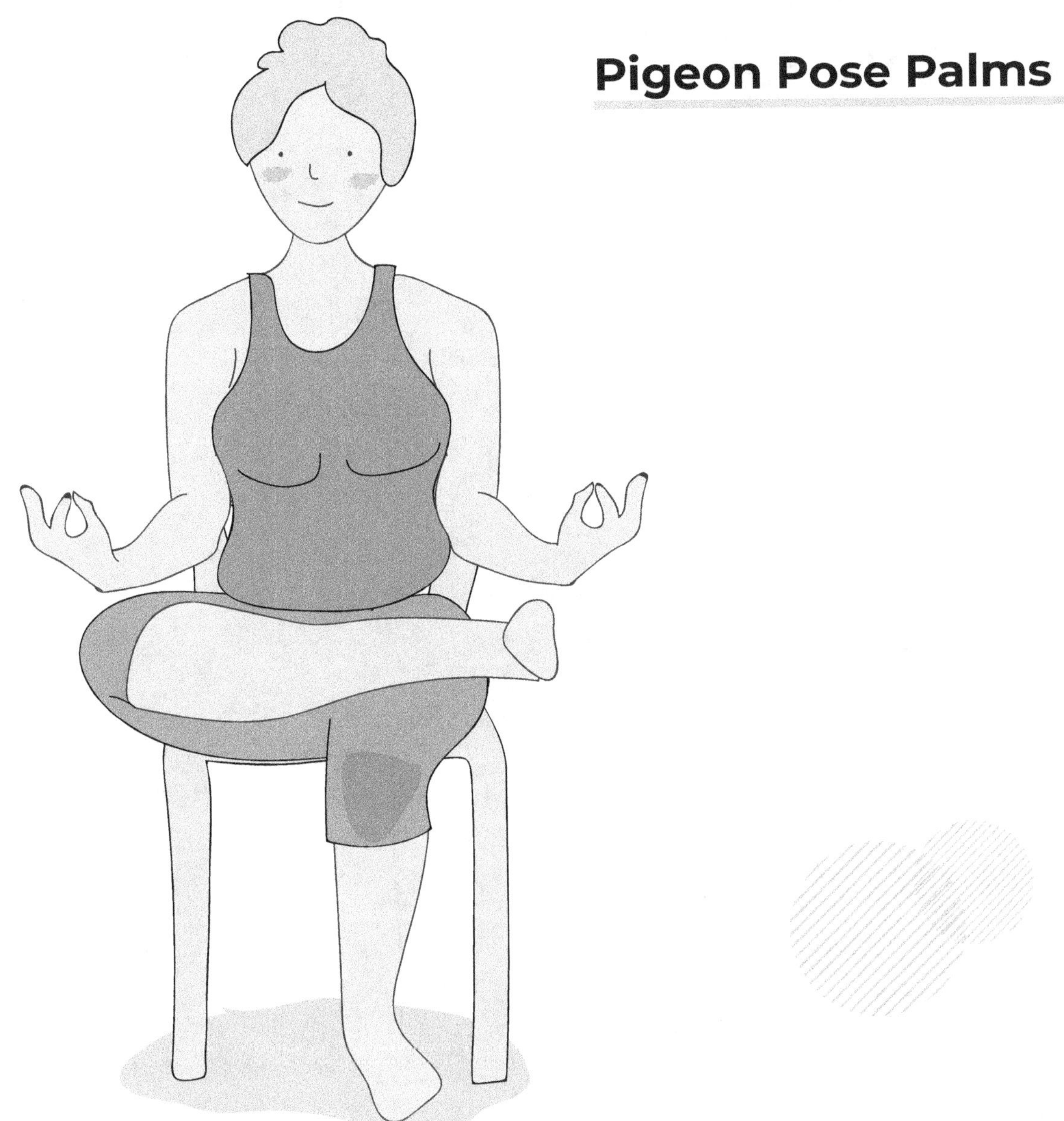

◈ Place one ankle on the opposite thigh, just above your knee.

◈ Bring the back of your hands to your leg, bringing your thumb and forefinger together.

◈ Keep your head aligned with your back and your gaze in front of you.

◈ Maintain this position for a few breaths while allowing your hips to stretch.

◈ Release slowly and take a few breaths.

◈ Repeat this exercise with the other side.

◈ When finished, return to the seated position listening to your body, for a few breaths.

Cat Pose Variation

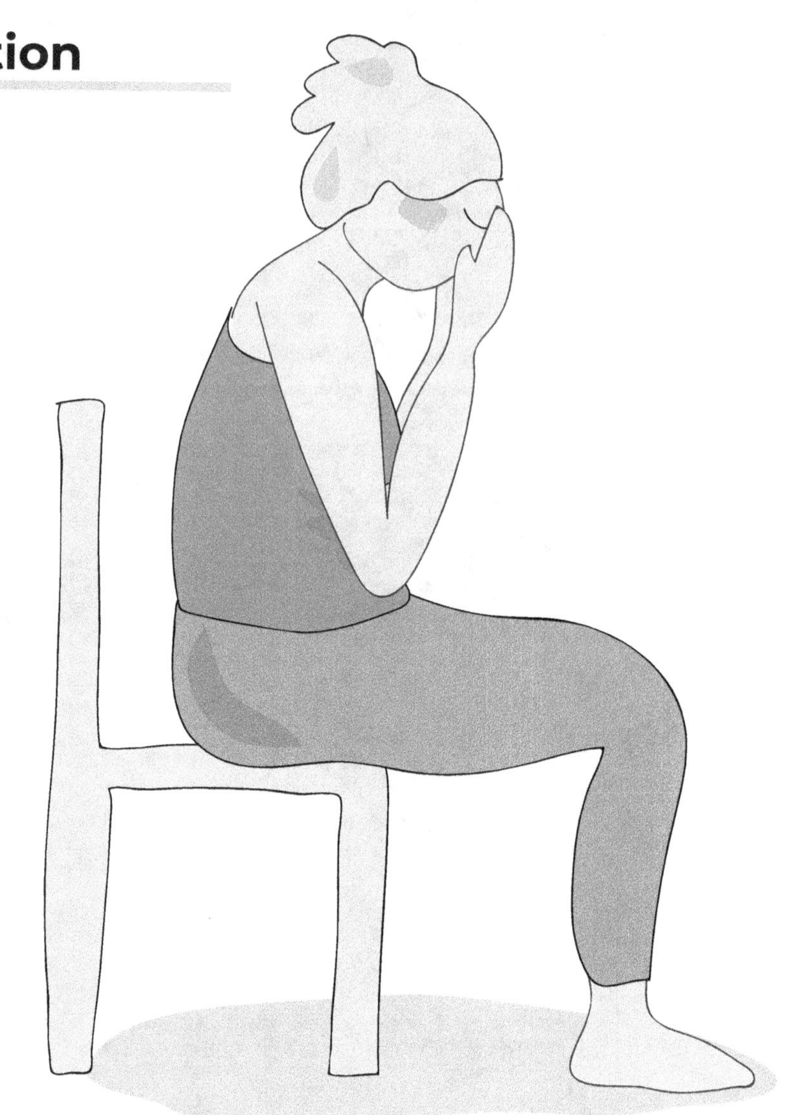

- ◈ While seated with your back straight, take a few deep breaths.
- ◈ Exhaling, arch your spine and bring your chin to your chest, pulling your shoulder blades away (cat pose).
- ◈ Cover your eyes with your hands to reduce external stimulation and create a sense of safety and comfort, which helps reduce stress and anxiety.

Covering your eyes can also help you rest and rejuvenate your vision. Relax completely for a few breaths.

This is a powerful way to promote relaxation, reduce stress, and complement the benefits of a yoga practice.

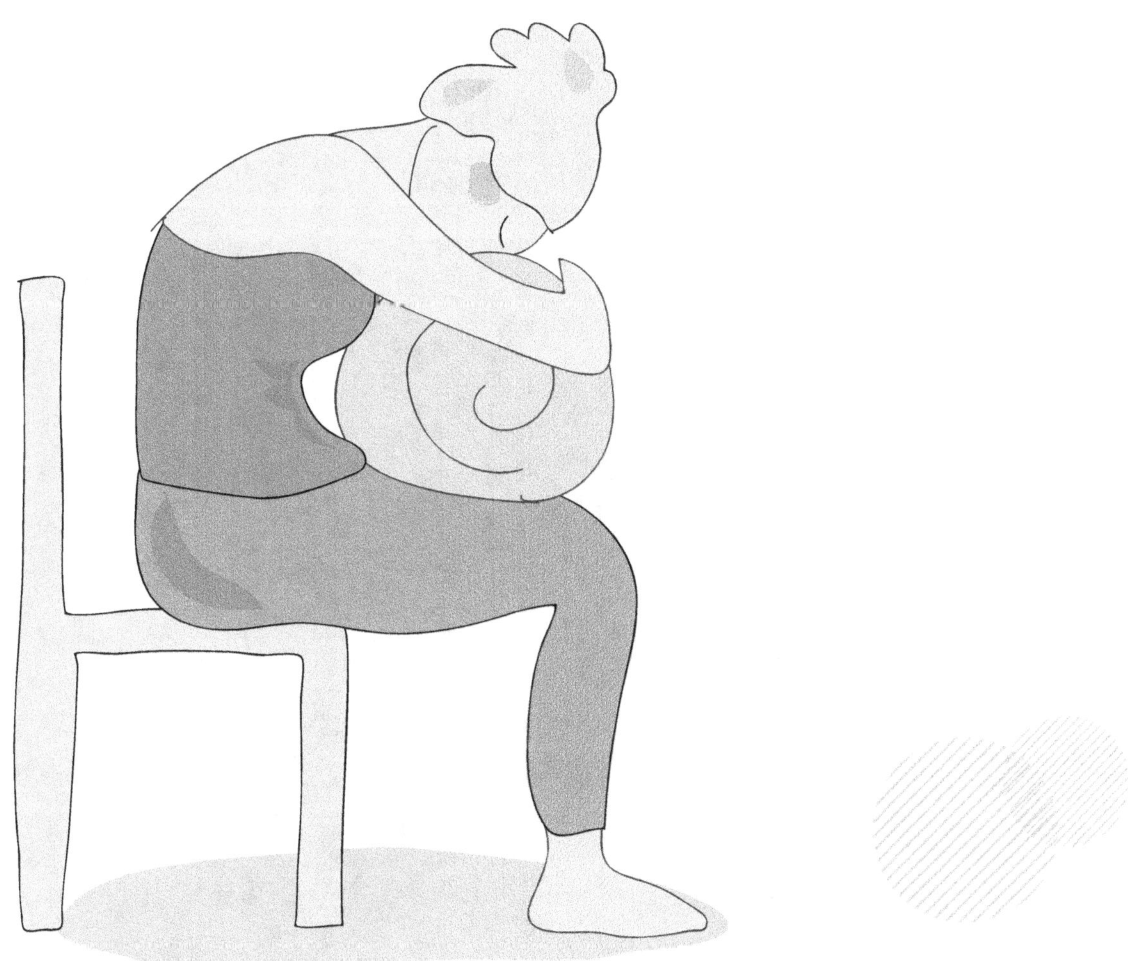

◈ While seated, take deep breaths.

◈ Place a pillow or a rolled-up blanket on your lap.

◈ Inhaling, place your arms on the pillow.

◈ Exhaling, let your torso rest on the pillow, leaving your whole body behind.

◈ Relax your shoulders, neck, head, back, and arms.

◈ Breathe in and feel the stretching of your back and neck.

◈ Gently release.

Forward Bend Deep

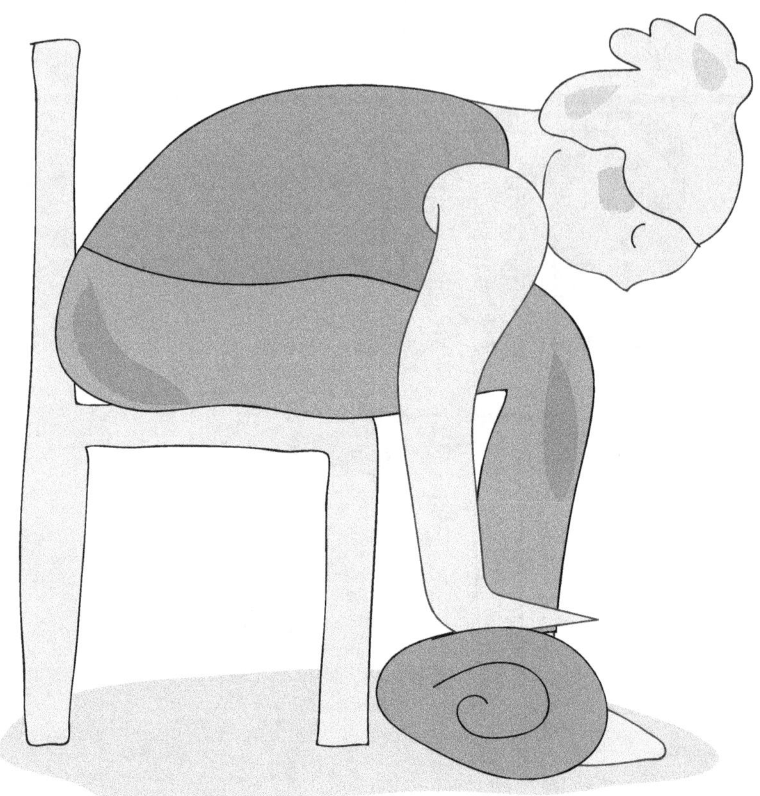

◈ While seated, breathe in deeply.

◈ Place a pillow or a rolled-up blanket on the floor near your feet.

◈ Exhaling, bend your upper body forward towards your thighs.

◈ Place your hands on the pillow and let your arms and shoulders relax.

◈ Breathe in and feel your back and neck lengthen.

◈ Gently return to the seated position.

This exercise promotes deep relaxation and encourages listening to your body, helping to alleviate stress and improve flexibility.

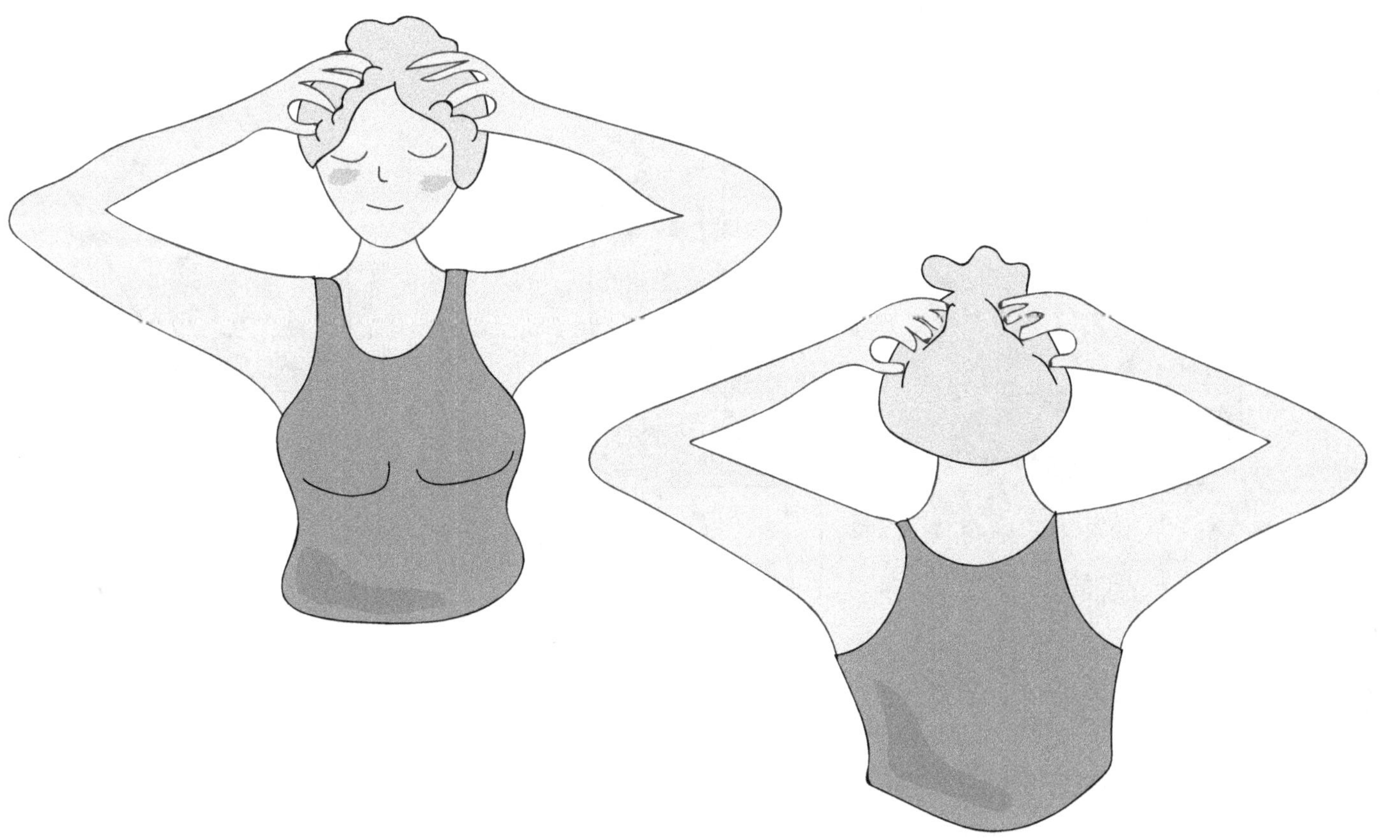

◈ Place your fingertips where your neck meets your head.

◈ Massage gently in circular movements without exerting excessive pressure.

◈ Move your fingertips up and down the scalp, massaging the entire area.

◈ Massage your temples and forehead with your fingertips, applying light pressure in circular movements.

◈ Continue for a few breaths, concentrating on the areas where you feel tension or discomfort.

◈ Breathe deeply and unwind. Massaging your head can be a great way to relieve tension and reduce stress.

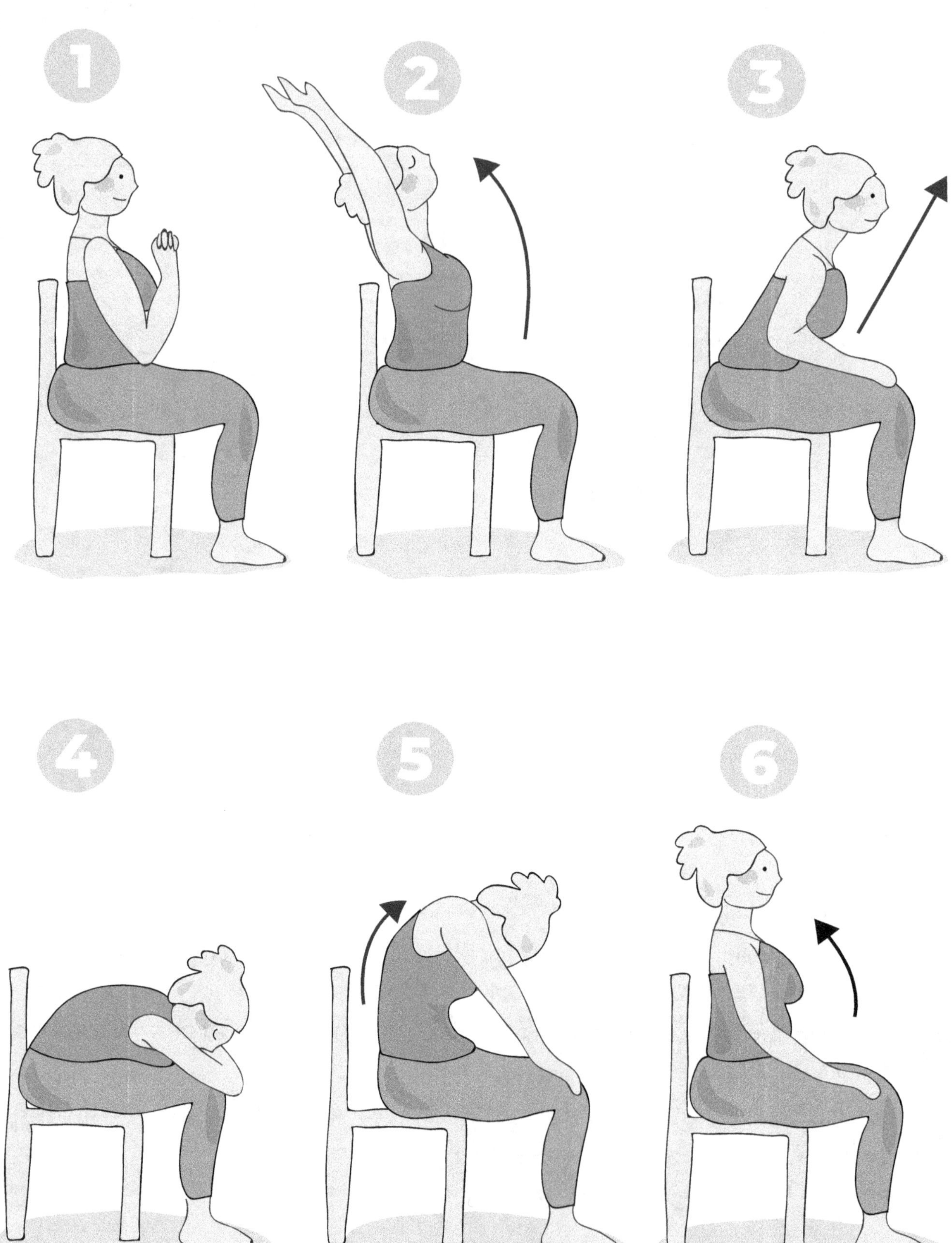

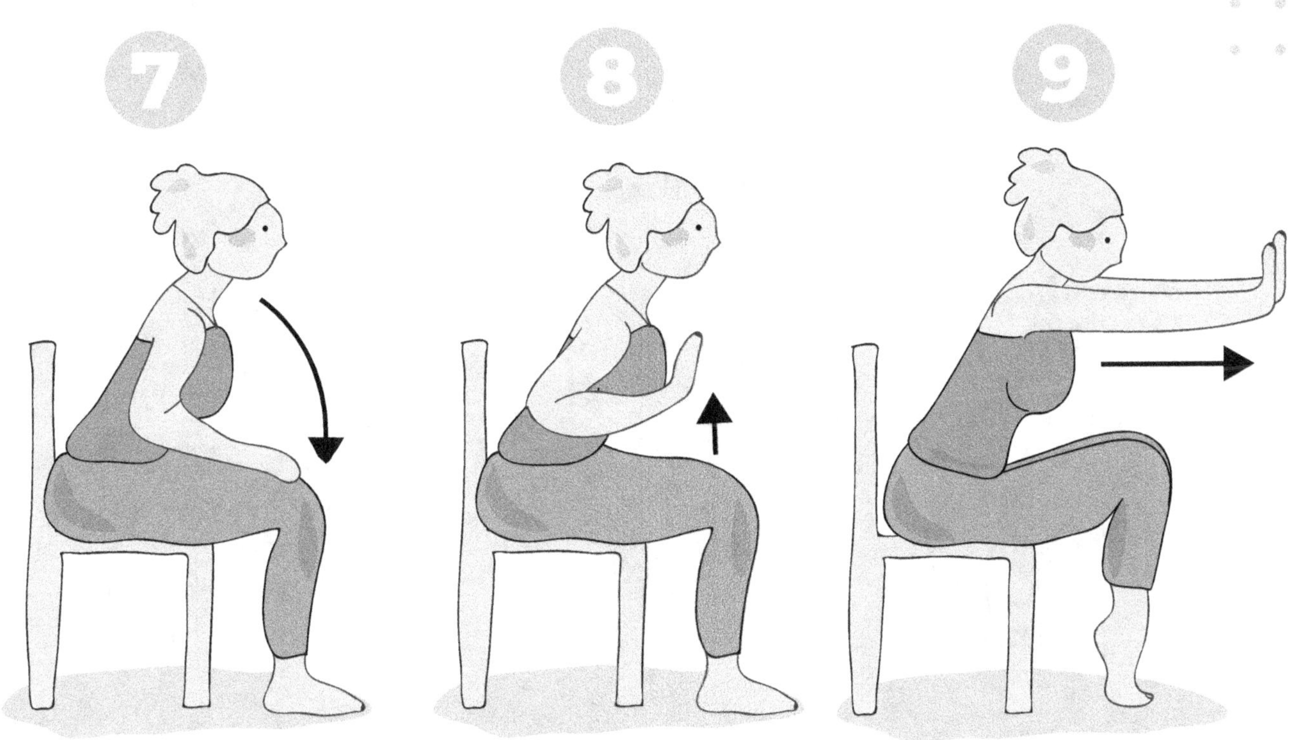

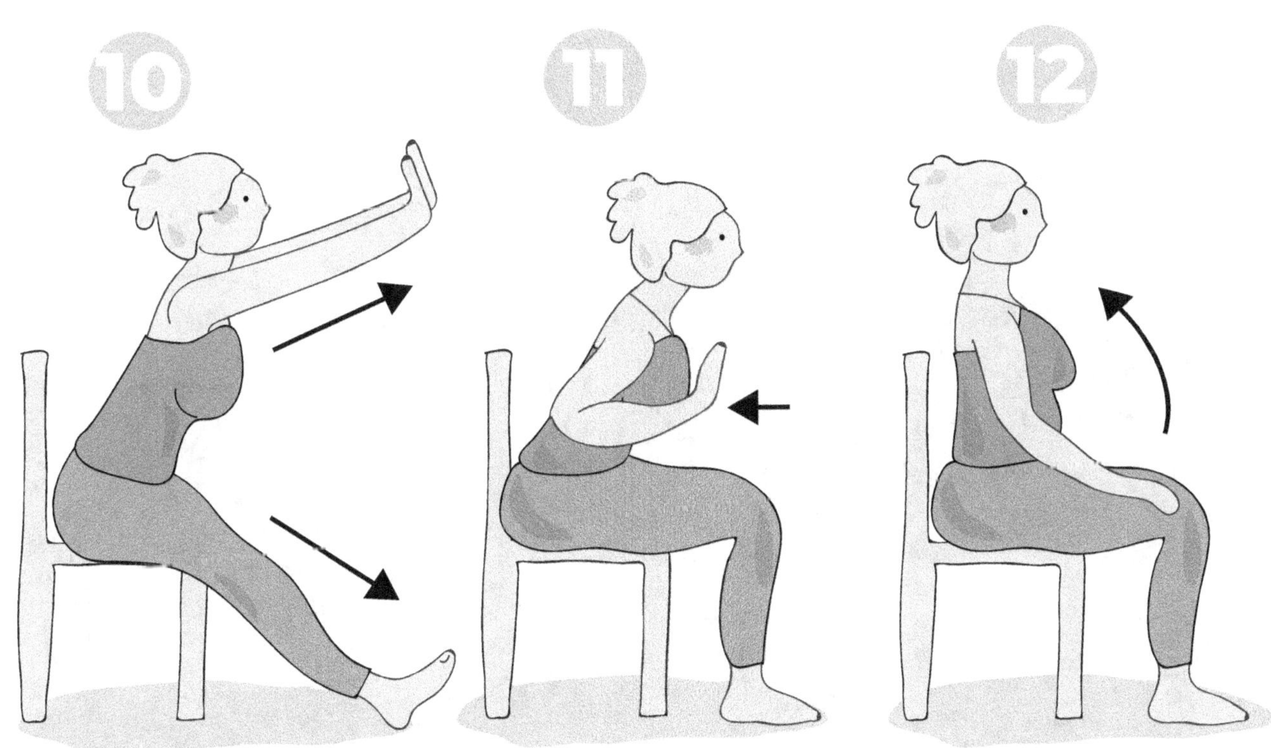

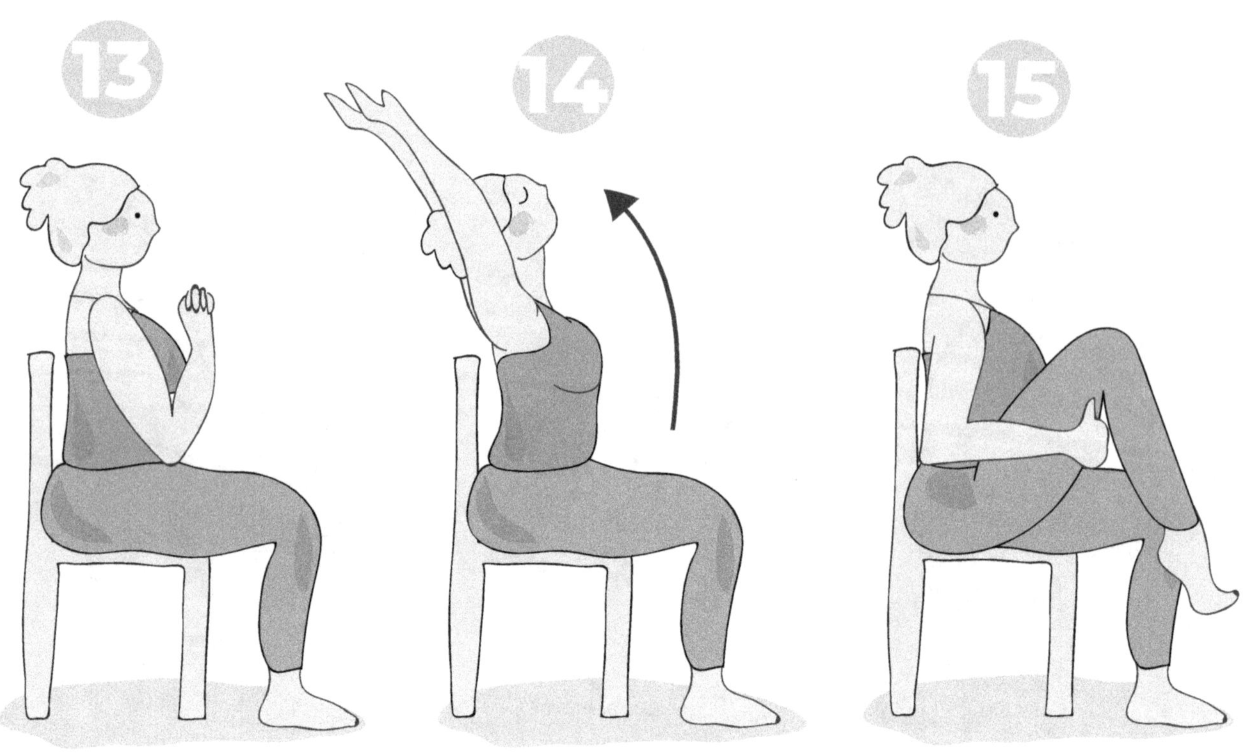

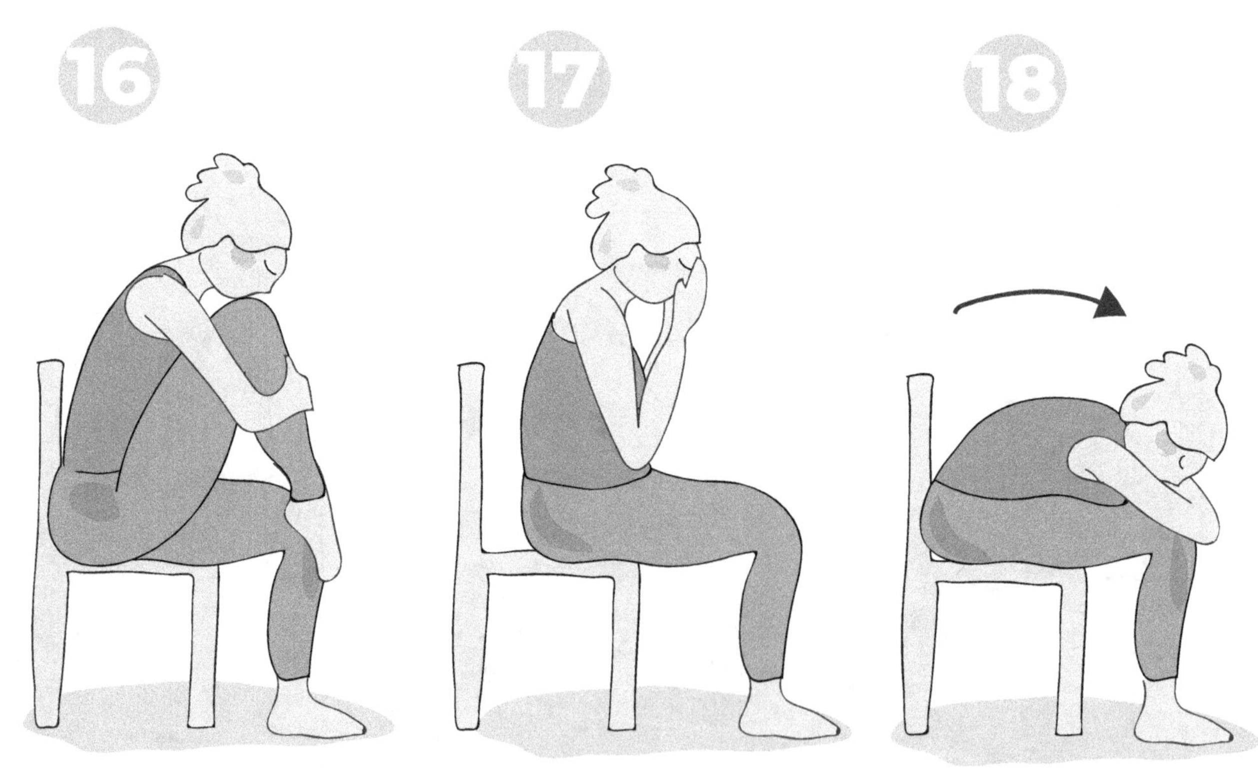

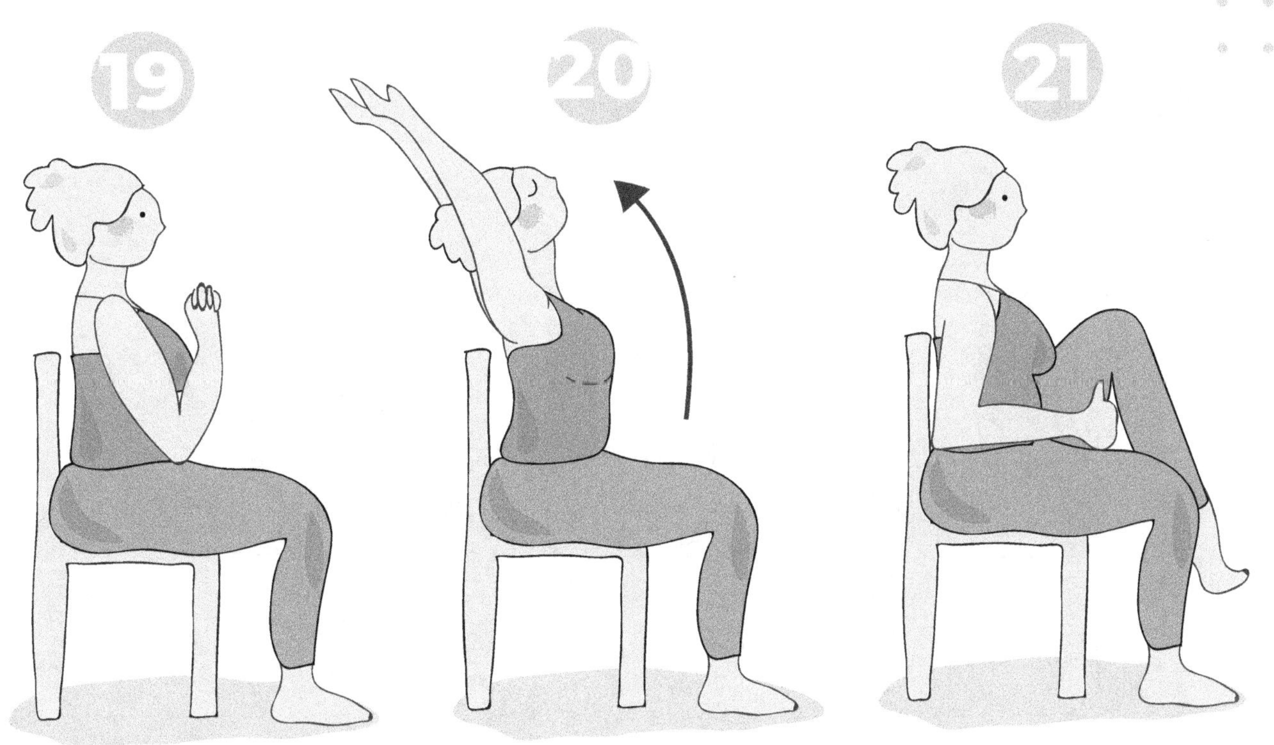

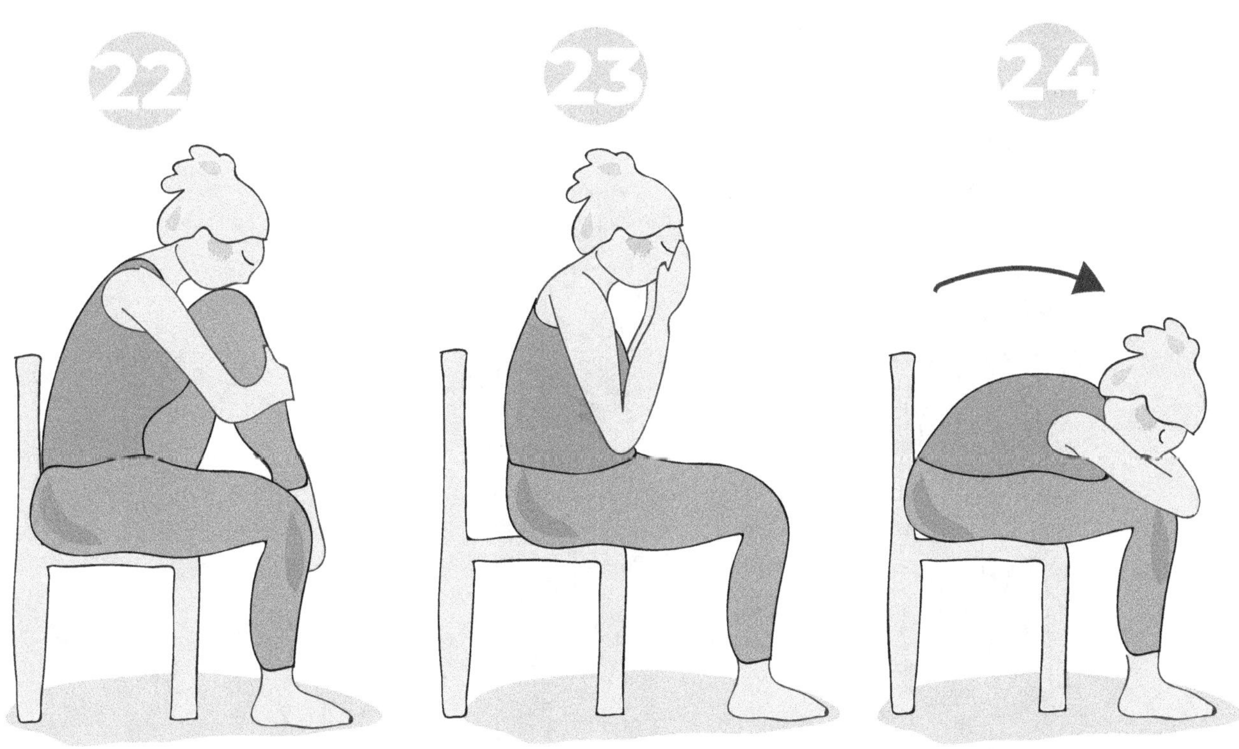

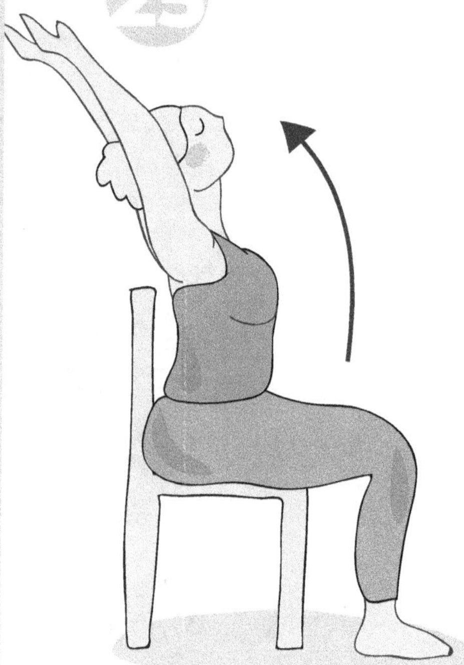

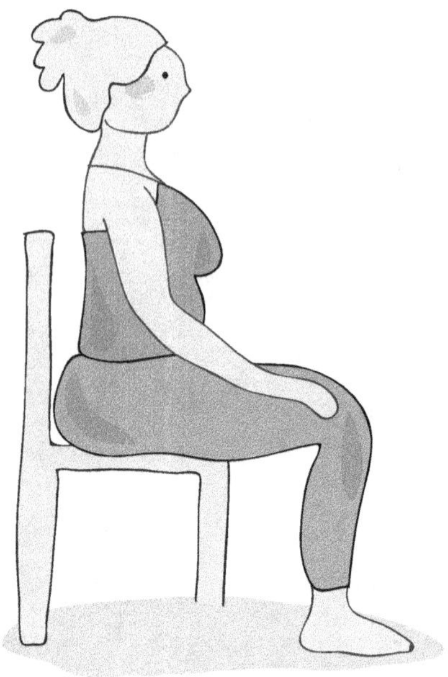

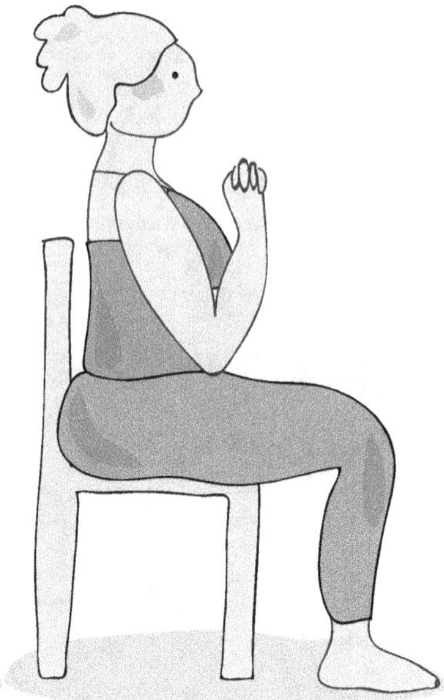

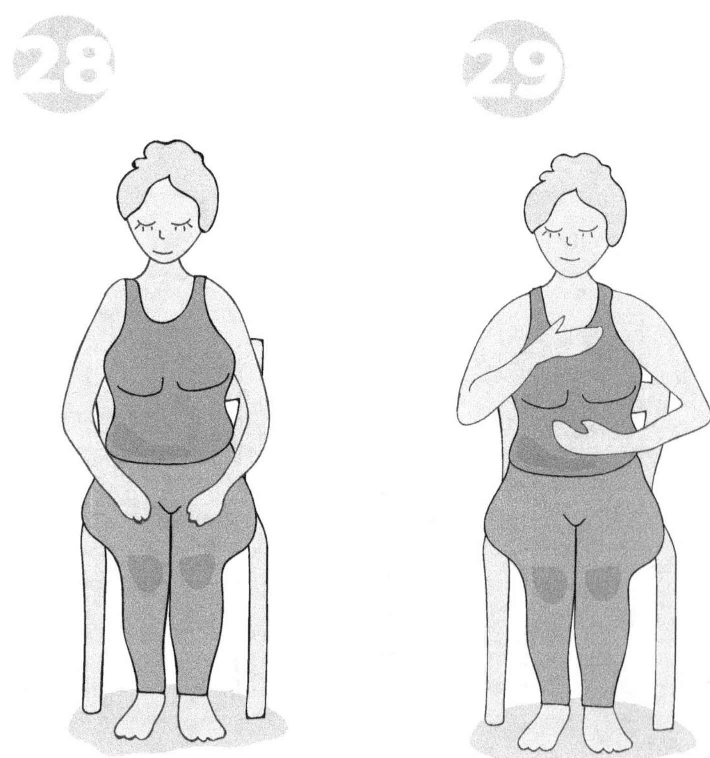

Meditation Pose: Chair Savasana

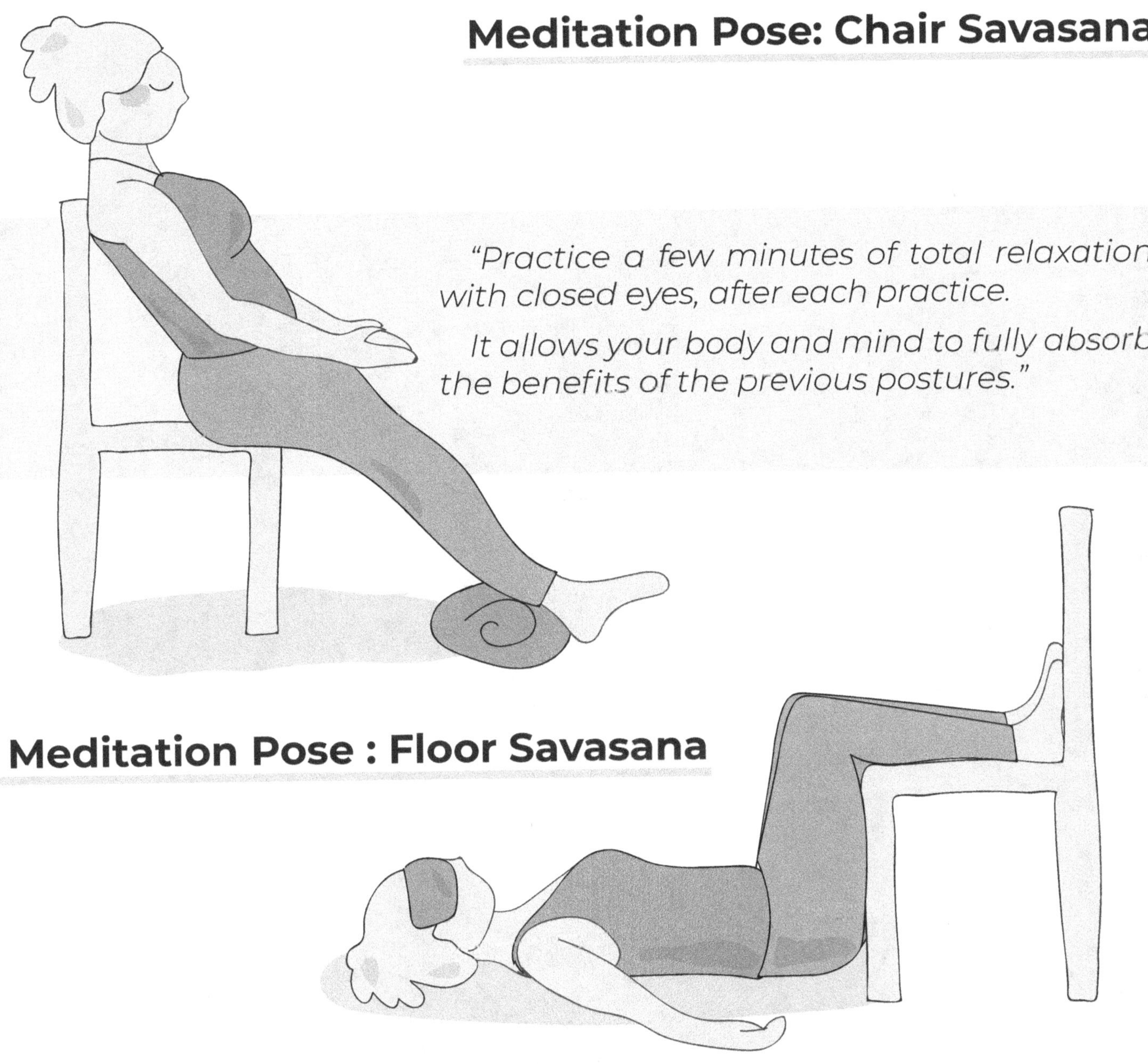

"Practice a few minutes of total relaxation with closed eyes, after each practice.

It allows your body and mind to fully absorb the benefits of the previous postures."

Meditation Pose : Floor Savasana

- ◈ Relax your body. Take a few moments to find a comfortable position and consciously relax your body.

- ◈ Focus. Feel your breath going in and out of your body.

- ◈ Practice non-judgmental awareness. When thoughts arise in your mind, simply welcome them, without judging them, then slowly bring your attention back to breathing.

- ◈ The goal of meditation is not to stop your thoughts from running, but to be aware of yourself, free of any judgment.

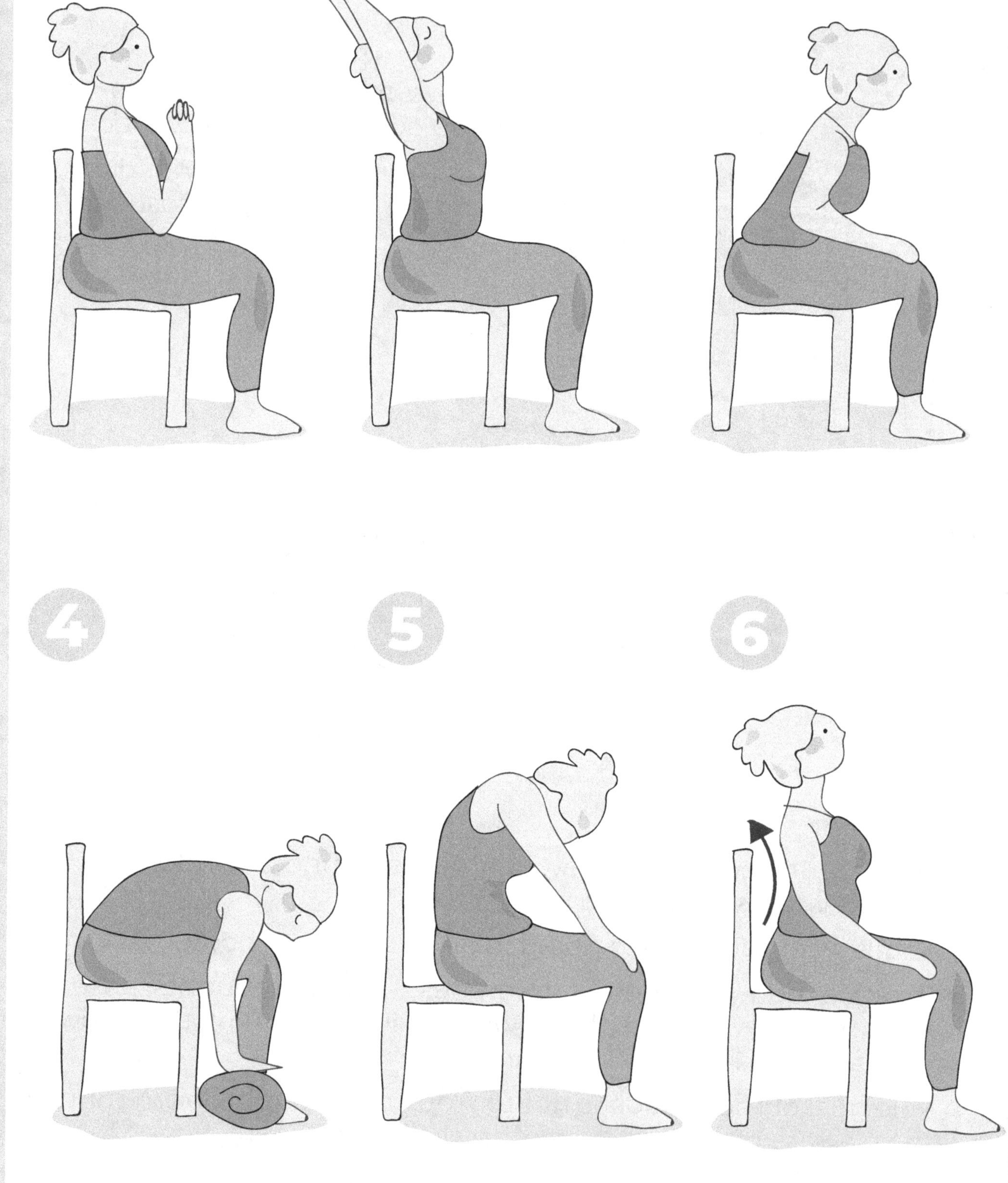

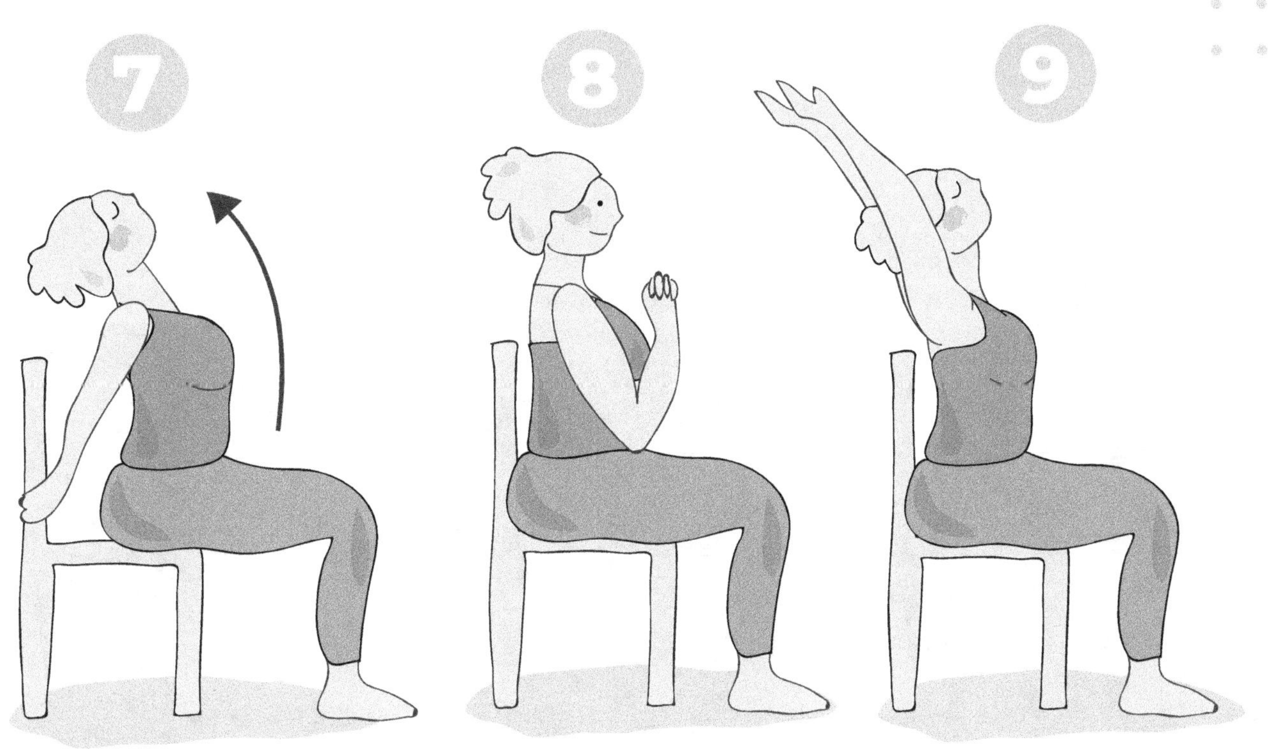

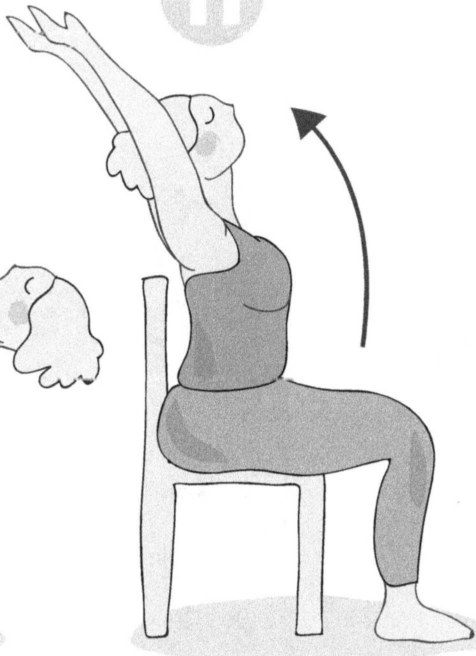

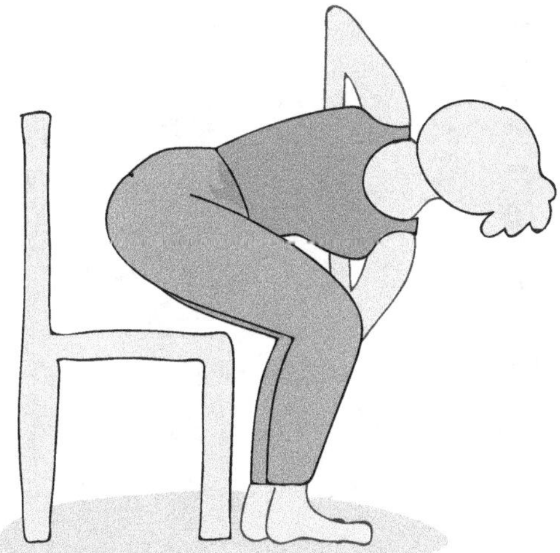

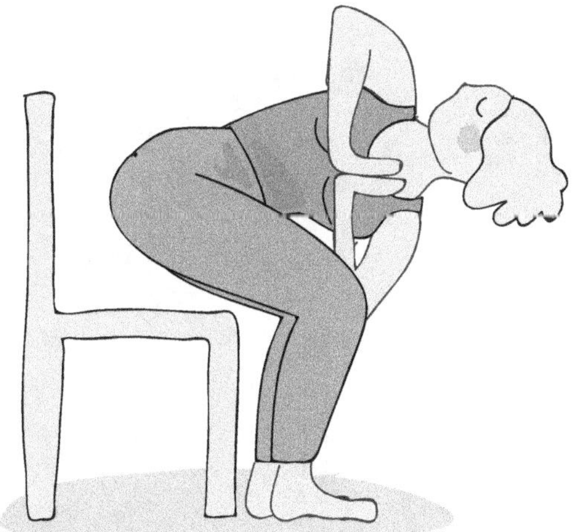

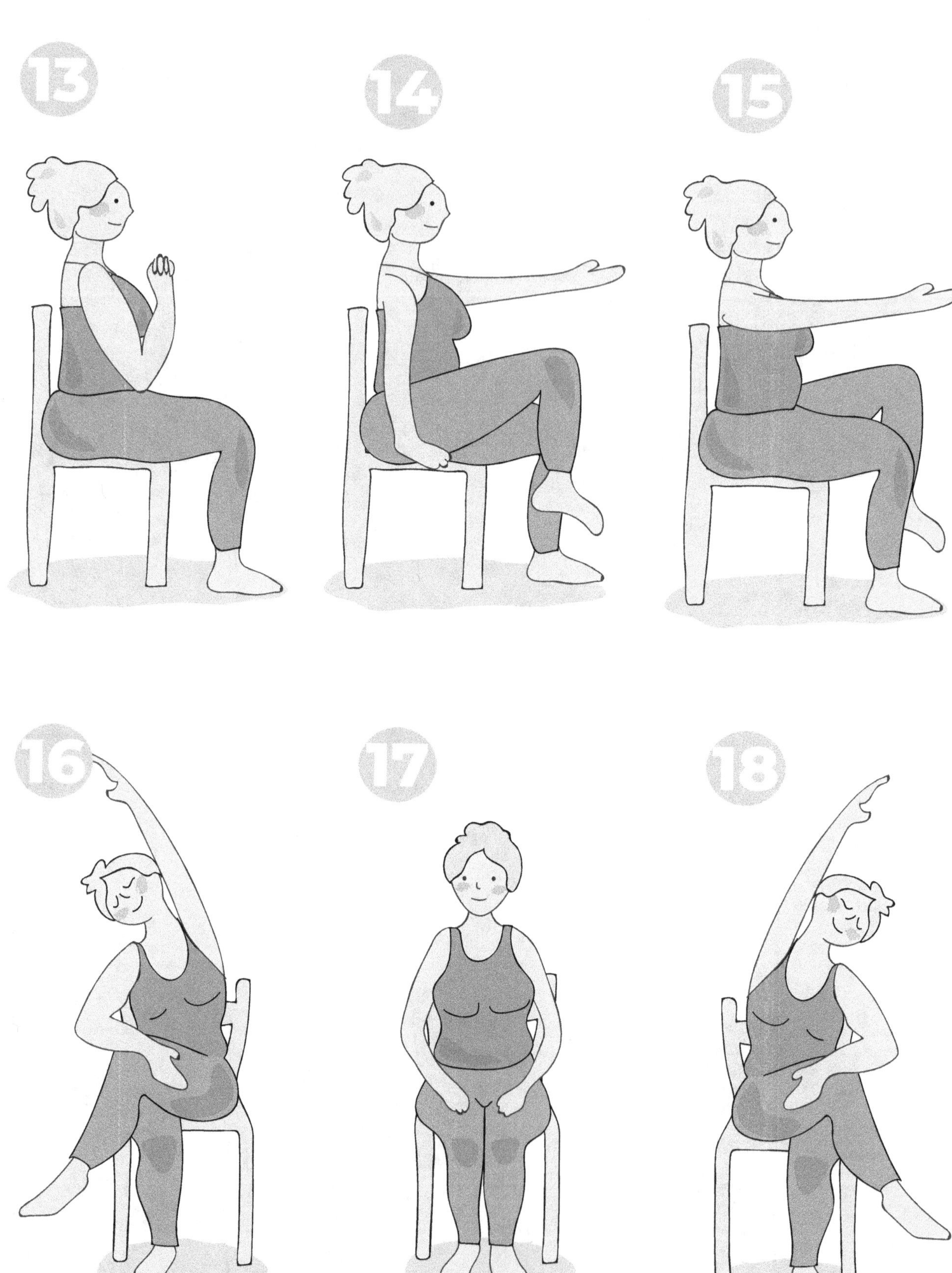

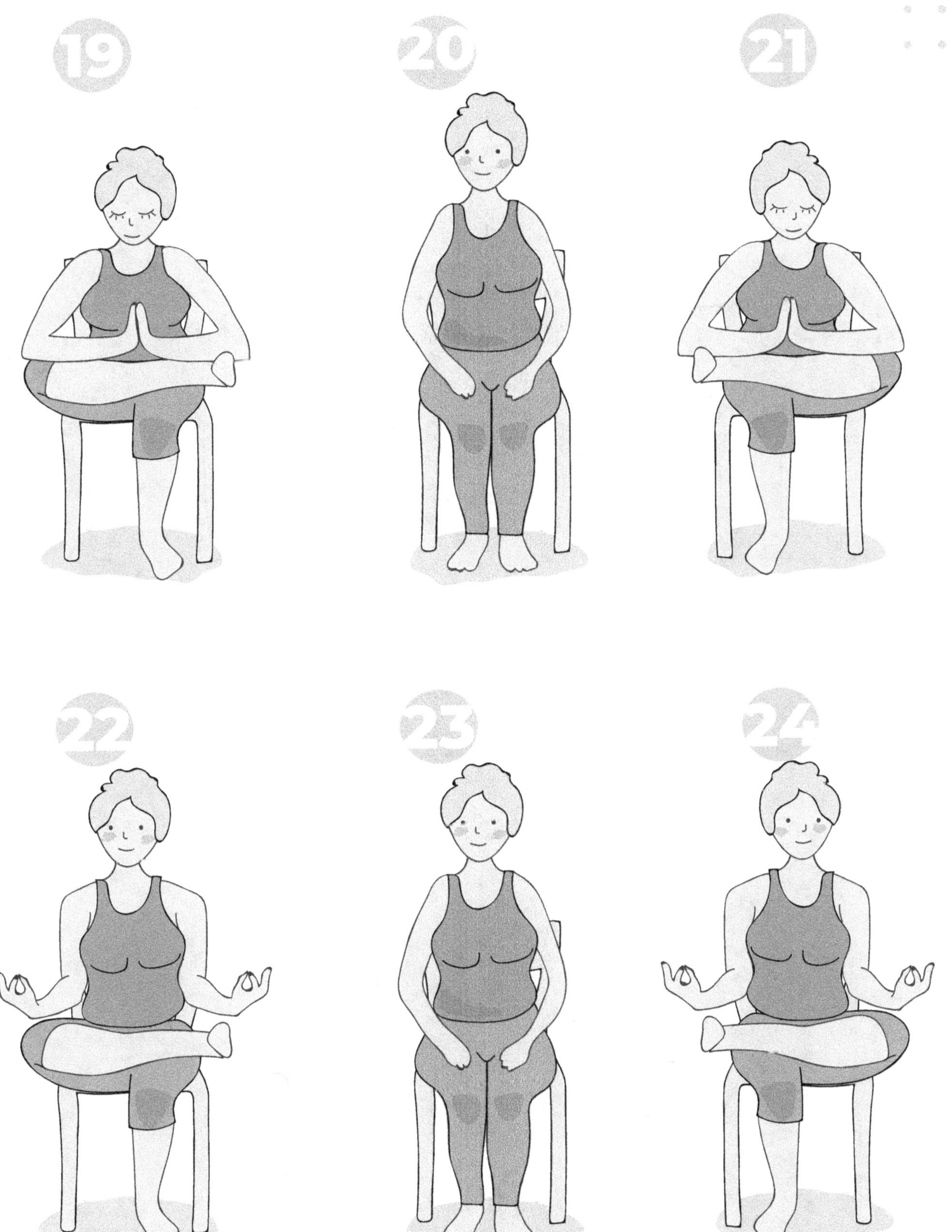

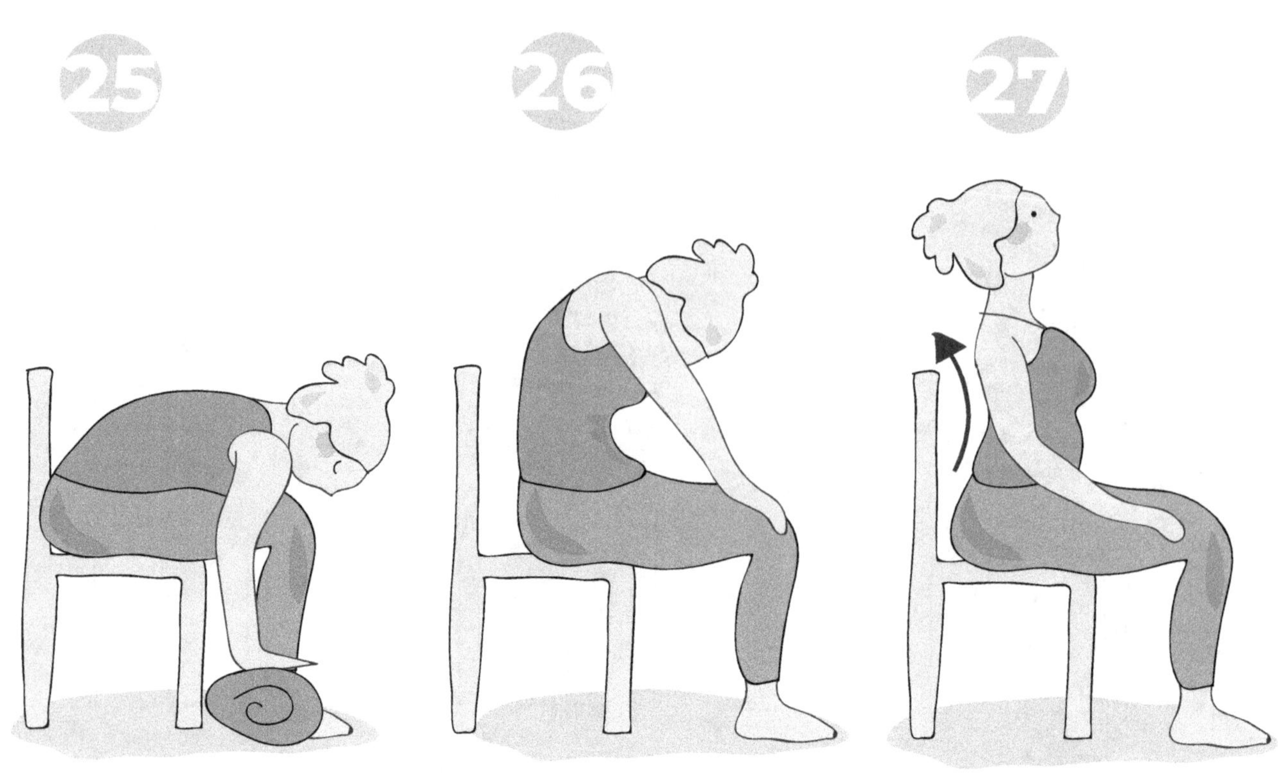

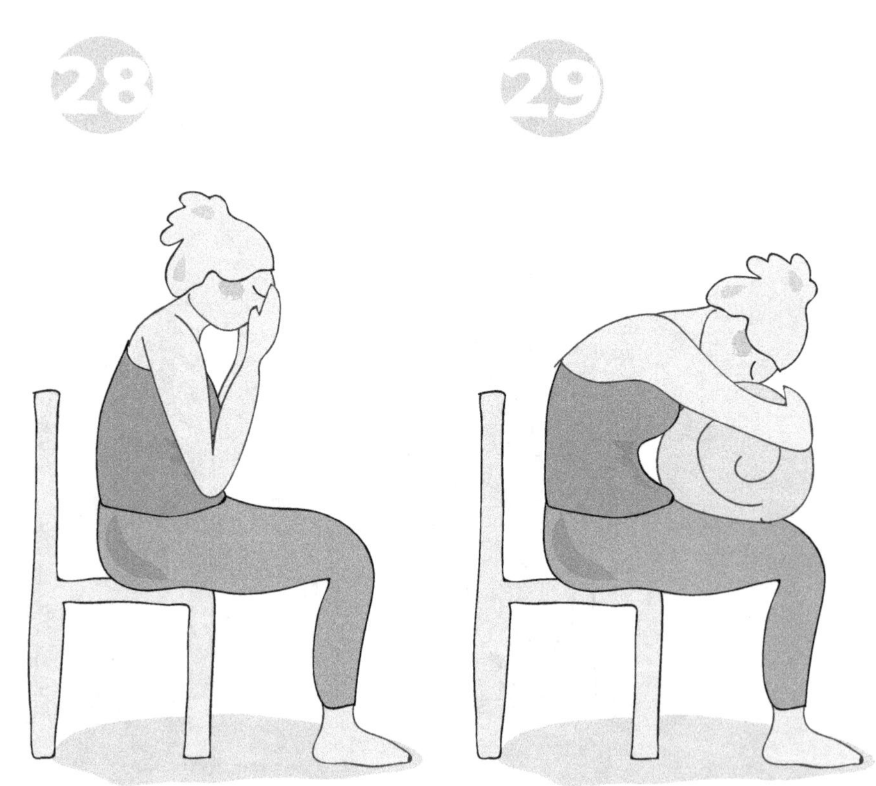

Yoga Nidra – Deep Relaxation to Sleep

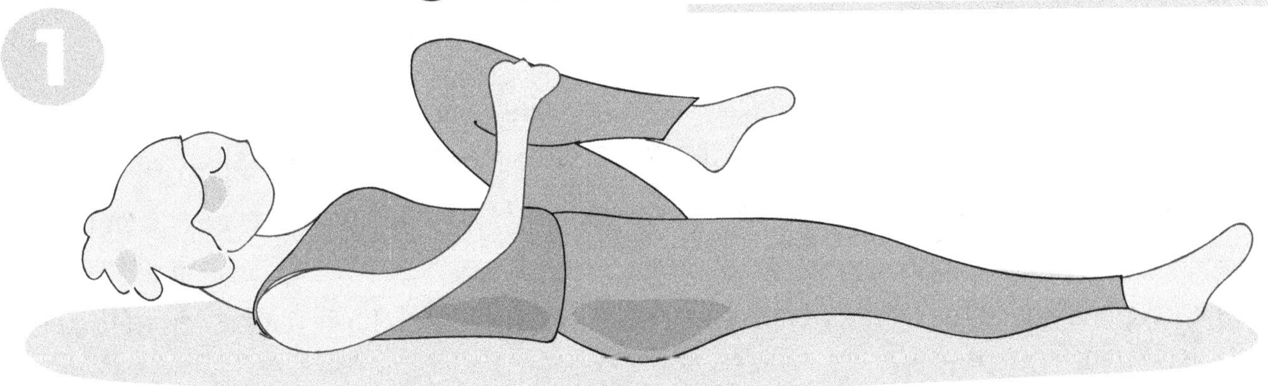

◈ While exhaling, gently bring your knee towards your forehead first with one leg and then with the other. Keep this position for a few breaths.

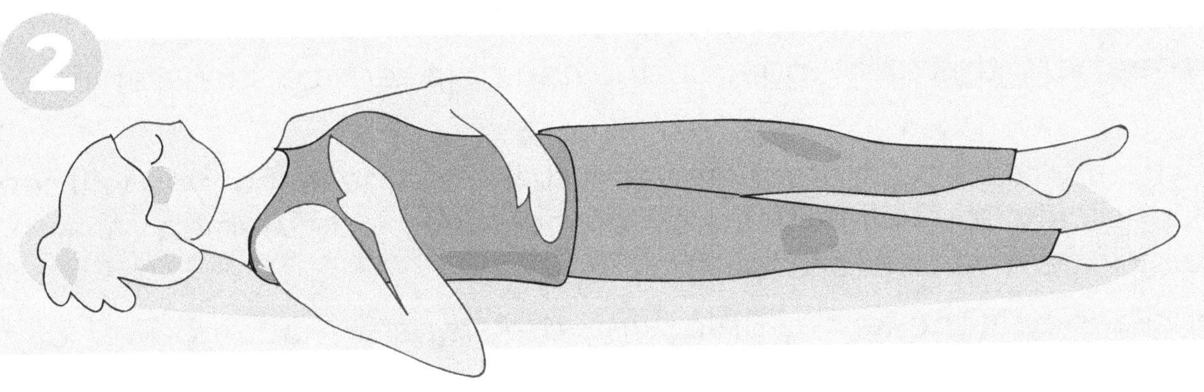

◈ Place the hands on your belly and chest and breathe in and out while feeling your chest and belly rise.

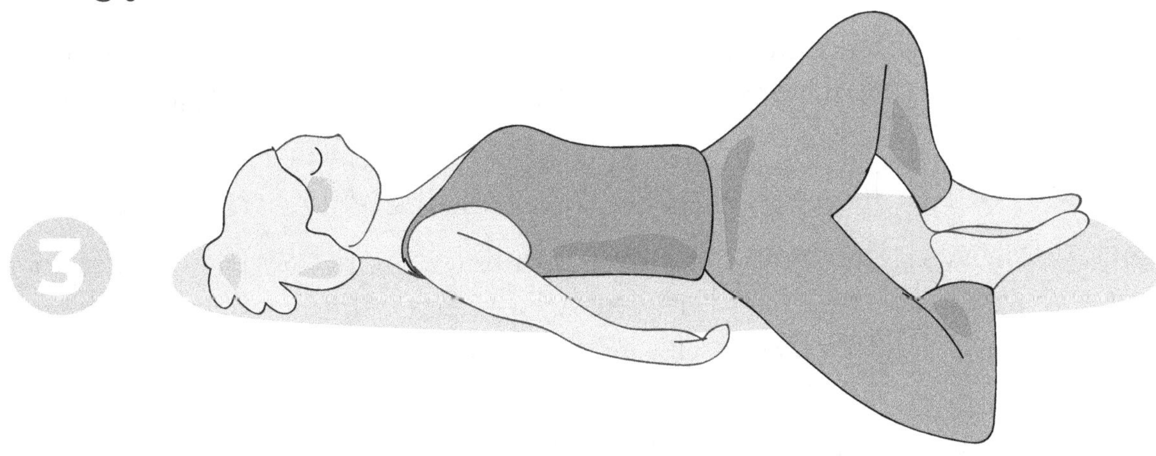

◈ Concentrate on your breathing. Try not criticizing your thoughts as they come to you.

DAILY ROUTINE

The chair yoga exercises suggested in this book can be performed on an as-needed basis for immediate relief from pain, tightness, or stiffness.

Establishing a daily routine is essential to getting the most out of practicing chair yoga.

Consistently performing the exercises can lead to more significant and long-lasting results.

By practicing the proposed 10-minute series daily, you will notice a significant improvement in your physical and psychological health.

These short series can improve flexibility, strength, and endurance, as well as increase your body and mind awareness.

Furthermore, this daily yoga routine can help reduce stress, anxiety, and insomnia.

The great thing about practicing this daily routine is that you will see the results quickly. You will notice a difference day by day, which will serve as a strong incentive to keep going.

"Consistency is the key to unlocking the transformative power of chair yoga in your life."

For maximum benefits, create a daily routine adapted to your needs and goals. Choose whether to practice in the morning or in the evening.

Have your chair and equipment ready to increase your motivation, especially at the beginning when you're still getting into the rhythm.

As with anything, chair yoga requires a little time and constant commitment, but unlike other activities, results will come immediately.

Constancy allows the body to gradually adapt to the positions and develop new skills. Repeating the exercises also allows you to strengthen neural connections, improve muscle memory, and increase precision and fluidity in your movements.

As you continue practicing, you'll find that your body starts craving the poses and exercises in the chair, making it easier and easier to practice each day.

Daily Routine Example for a More Vibrant Life

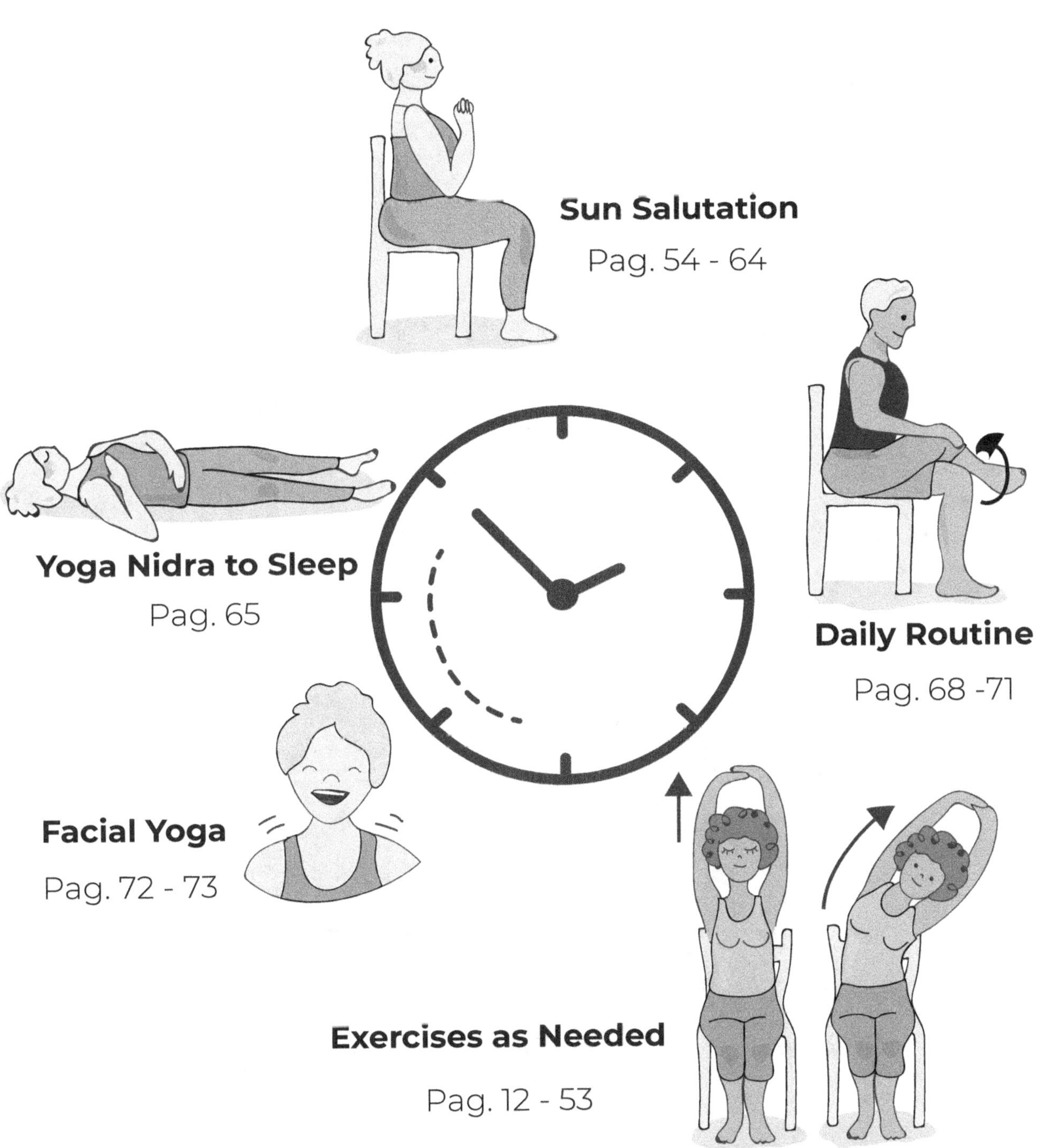

① Breathing Exercise
Duration 2 min

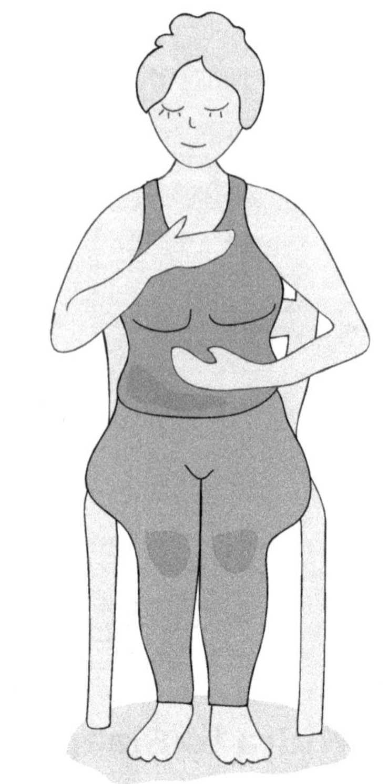

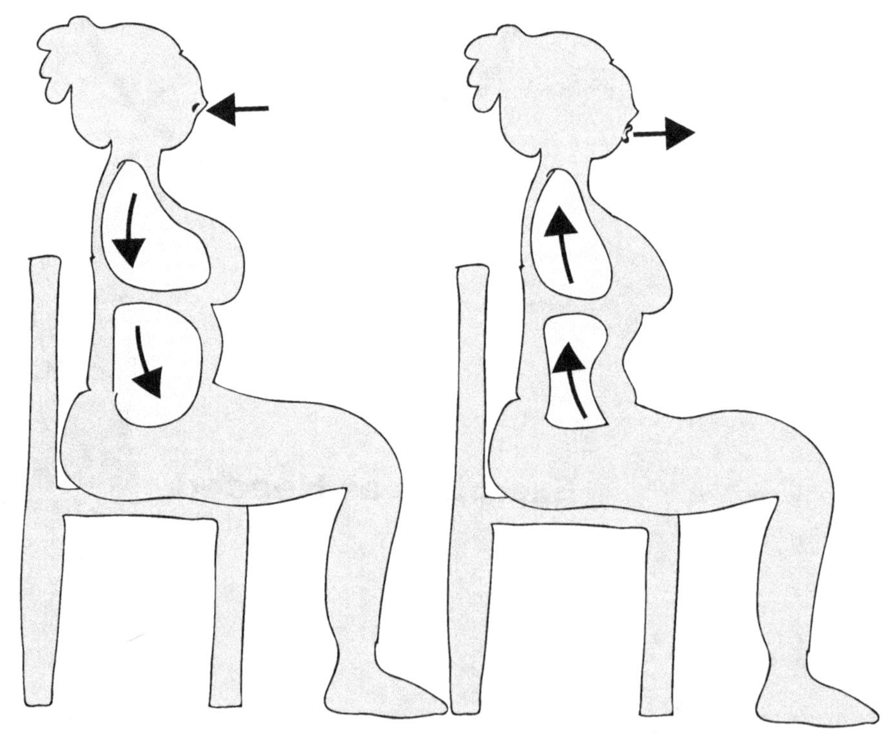

Warm-Up Exercises
Duration 2 min

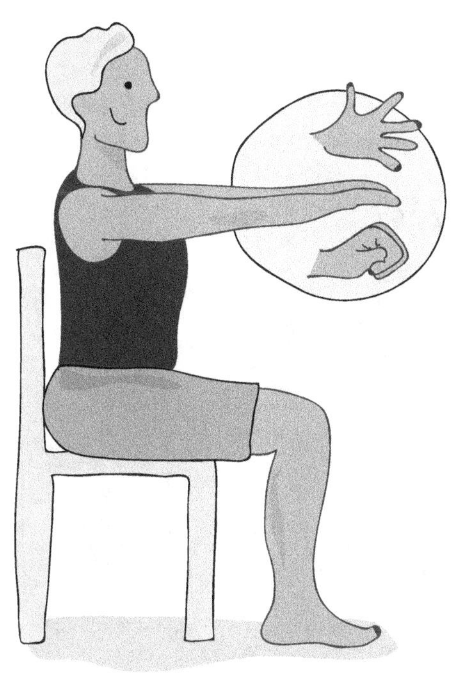

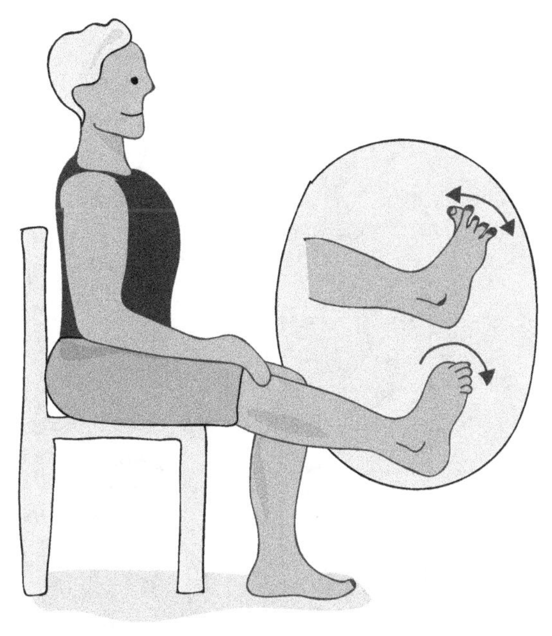

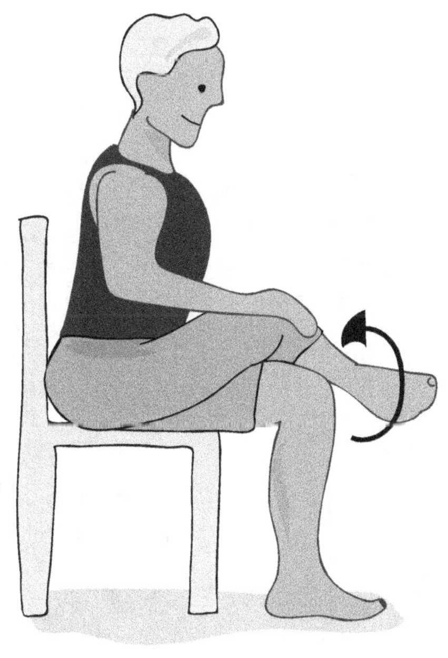

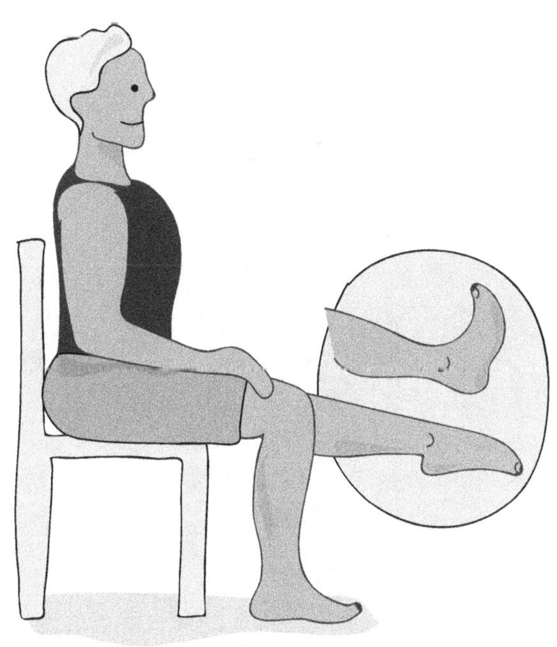

3

Yoga Practice
Duration 4 min

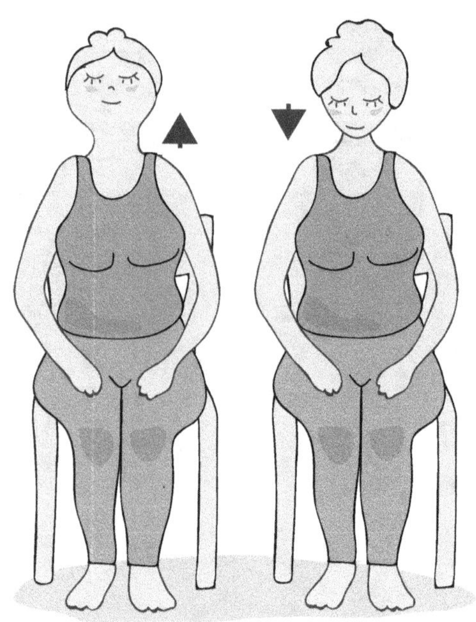

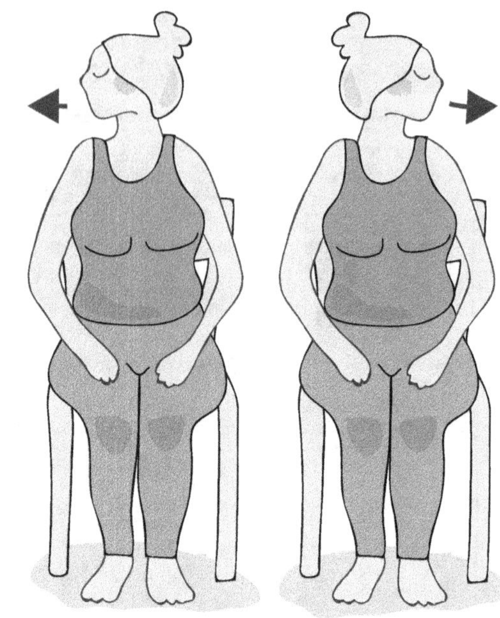

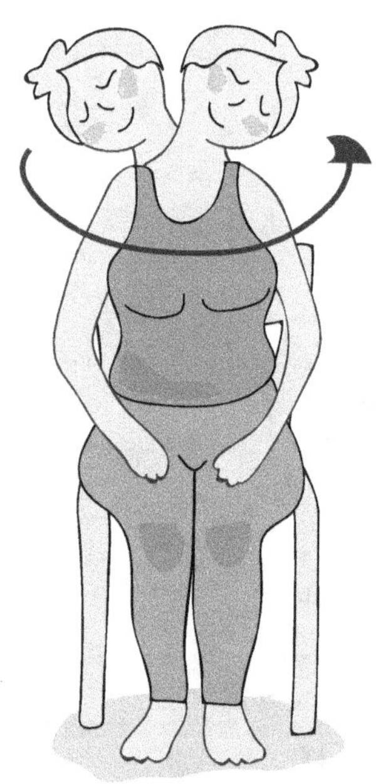

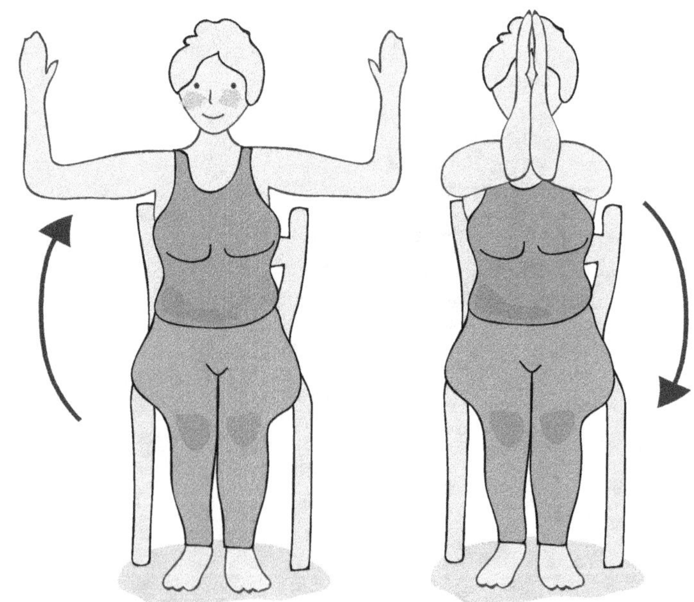

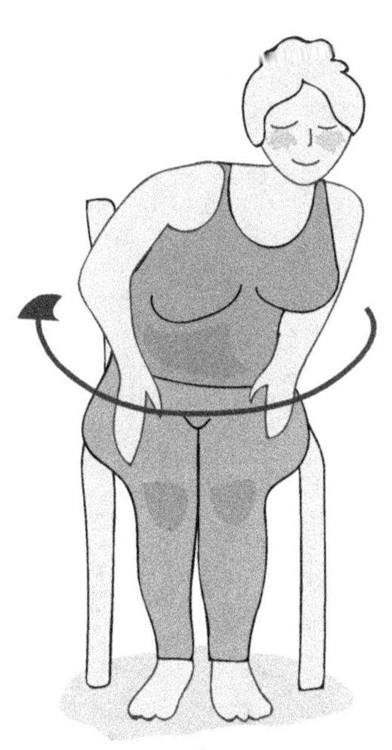

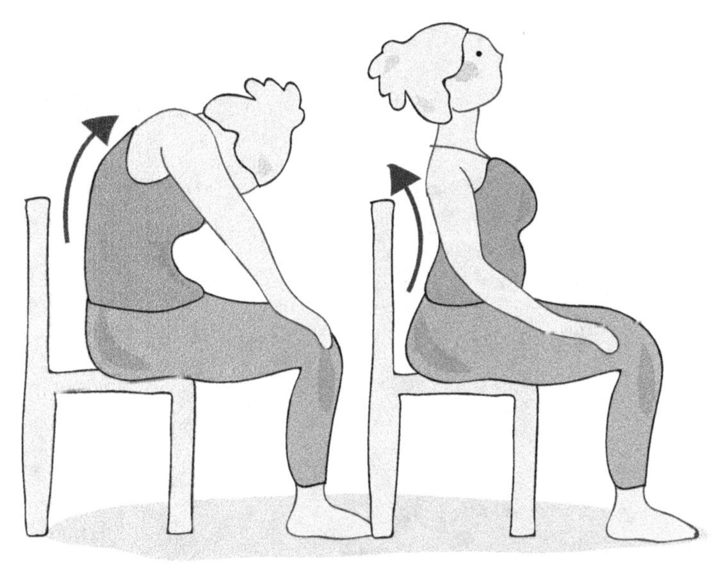

4. Defatigue and Meditation
Duration 2 min

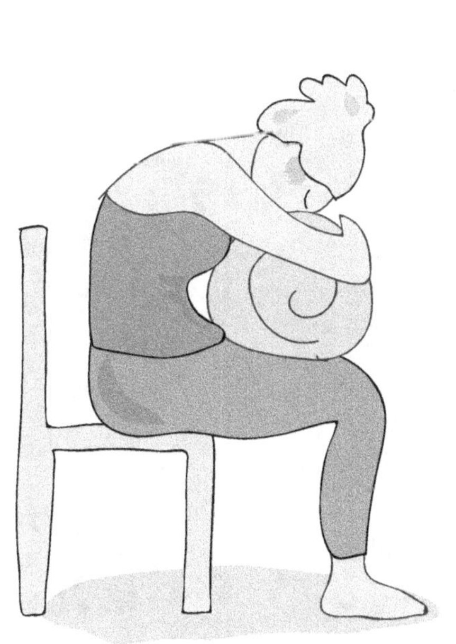

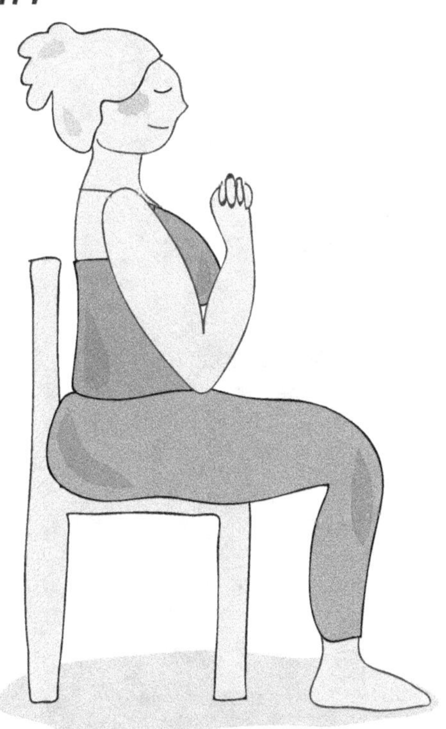

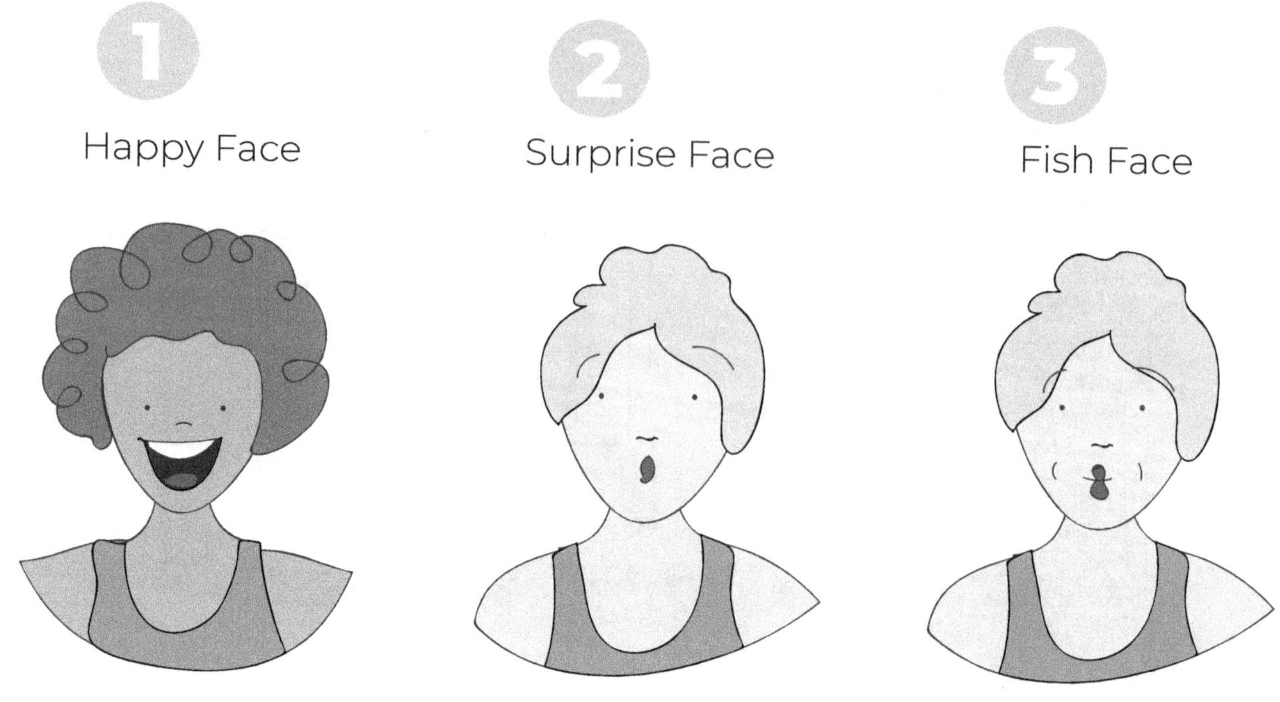

Facial yoga is a natural and effective way to maintain healthy, young-looking skin while promoting relaxation and reducing stress.

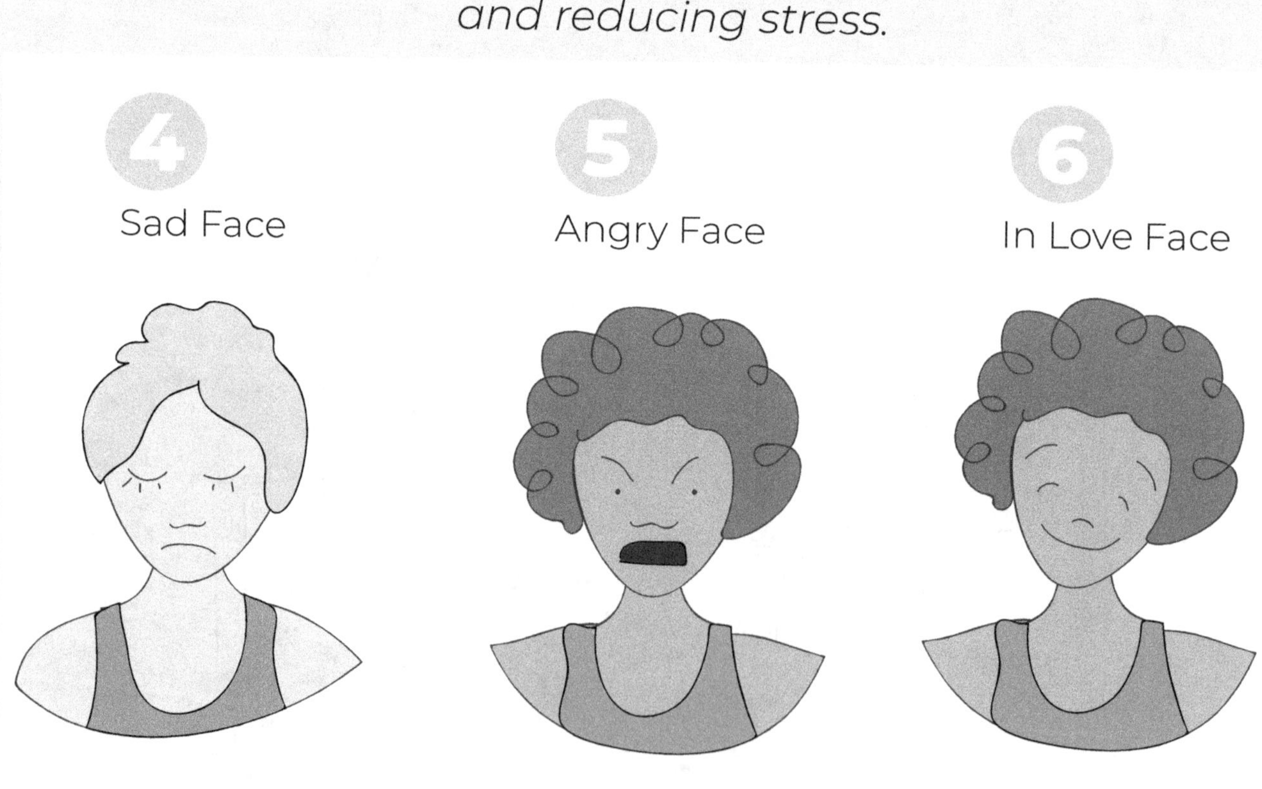

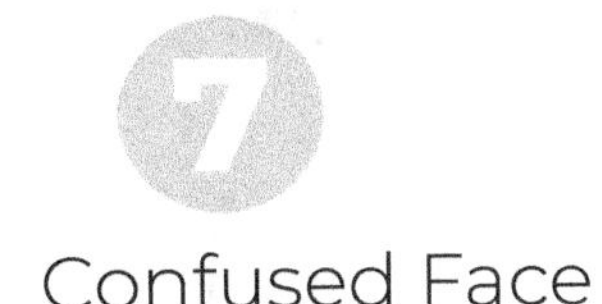

Confused Face

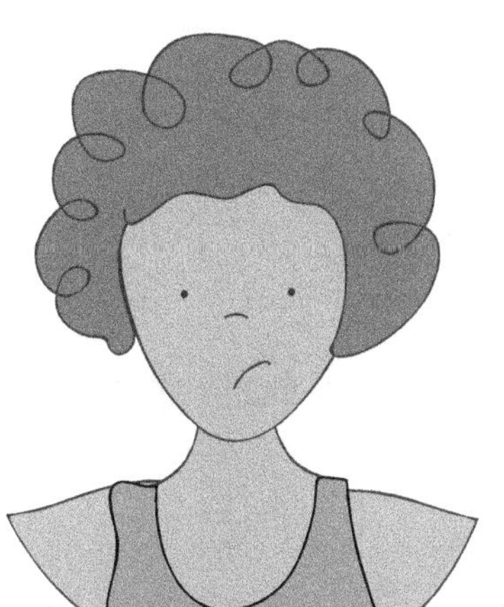

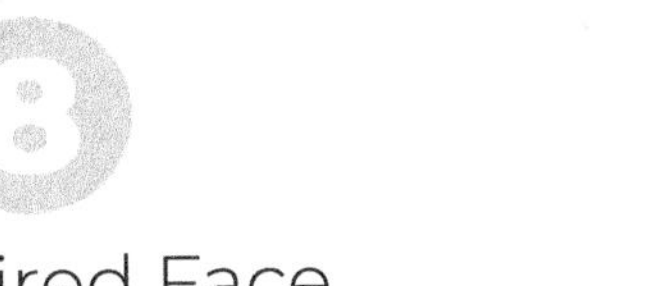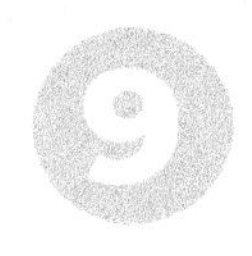

Tired Face

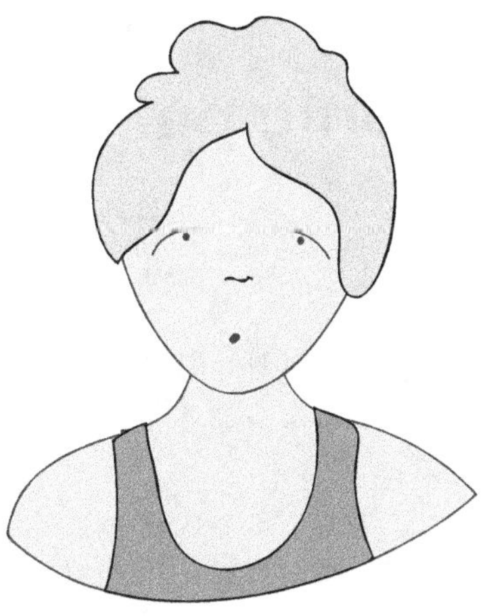

Yawn Face

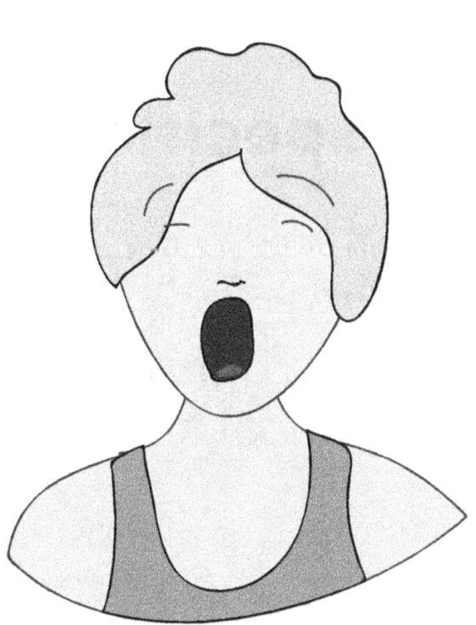

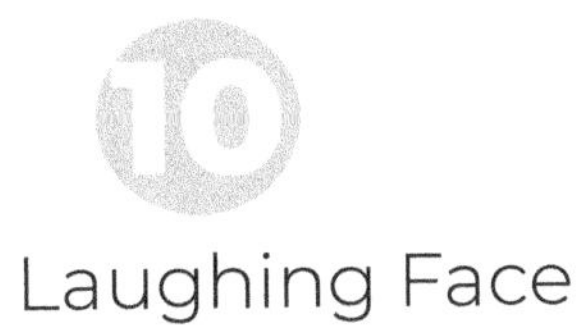

Laughing Face

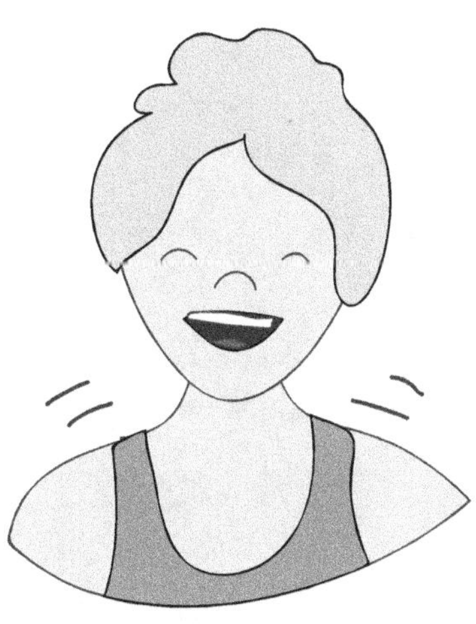

◈ *Repeat the sequence several times a day.*

◈ *Relax your facial muscles while reducing wrinkles.*

◈ *Improve your blood circulation, relieve tension, and boost your self-confidence, and most of all, enjoy it!*

CONCLUSION - Healing Through Yoga

If you are dealing with a specific health issues, there are tailor-made exercises to help you with your condition.

Specific and chronic pain

IMPORTANT NOTE:

This manual is in no way intended as a substitute for specific medical care.

Pain is a common issue among seniors due to conditions like arthritis, osteoporosis, and other chronic illnesses, which can limit your mobility and quality of life. However, chair yoga has been suggested as a potential complementary therapy to alleviate chronic pain and improve mobility for seniors.

◈ Arthritis 20, 29, 30, 37, 54

◈ Back pain 16, 25, 26, 28, 33

◈ Feet pain 20, 29, 30, 41

◈ Fibromyalgia 54, 60, 72

◈ Headaches 12, 50, 51, 53, 72

◈ Hand pain 20, 36, 37, 53

◈ Neck pain 17, 18, 19, 21, 26

◈ Neuropathy 50, 60 72

◈ Osteoporosis 18, 19, 21, 23, 24 38, 42

◈ Peripheral artery disease 54

◈ Poor posture 12, 16, 22, 24, 31

◈ Spondylosis 54

◈ Trigeminal neuralgia 12, 35, 53, 73

Reduced balance and mobility

People with reduced mobility and balance can experience negative outcomes such as decreased independence, social isolation, increased risk of falling, and reduced quality of life. Nevertheless, chair yoga can be a valuable method for improving your physical function and mobility. By practicing chair yoga, you can enhance flexibility, balance, strength, and range of motion, reducing the risk of falling and improving your overall physical health.

◈ Alzheimer's disease 13, 23, 32, 37, 72

◈ Pulmonary disease 12, 13, 14, 15, 16

◈ Incontinence 16, 42, 44, 45, 46, 47

◈ Multiple sclerosis (MS) 54, 60

◈ Parkinson's disease 68

Memory and Concentration problems

People with memory and concentration problems may have difficulties completing everyday tasks and may feel less independent, leading to a lower quality of life. Practicing chair yoga can be an effective way to improve cognitive function. Through physical exercise, chair yoga can increase blood flow to the brain, stimulate the nervous system, and enhance cognitive function.

◈ Anxiety and sadness 12, 13, 16, 59, 62

◈ Sleep apnea 65

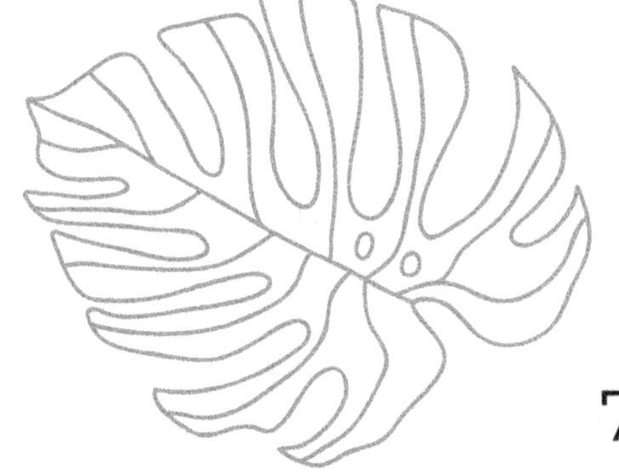

About the Author

Luna Lotus discovered the benefits of yoga in her mid 40s when she was working as a social worker and started having back problems.

After years of dealing with the stress and the emotional toll of her job, she found that practicing yoga helped her manage her anxiety and find inner peace.

Over time, Luna became passionate about sharing the benefits of yoga with others, especially older adults who may not have realized that yoga is accessible to them.

She trained to become a yoga instructor and focused on developing classes and programs that were safe and appropriate for seniors from all walks of life.

Yoga is not about competition, but about progress.

As Luna continued to practice and teach yoga, she noticed how it positively impacted her own physical and mental health as she aged.

She began to specialize in yoga for seniors and became a sought-after instructor in her community.

Luna eventually decided to start writing about yoga for seniors, hoping to reach a wider audience with her message about the transformative power of yoga.

Her writing includes tips and advice for older adults looking to start practicing yoga, as well as stories from her own experience and those of her students.

Luna stays committed to educating elders worldwide about the advantages of yoga and continues to practice it every day.

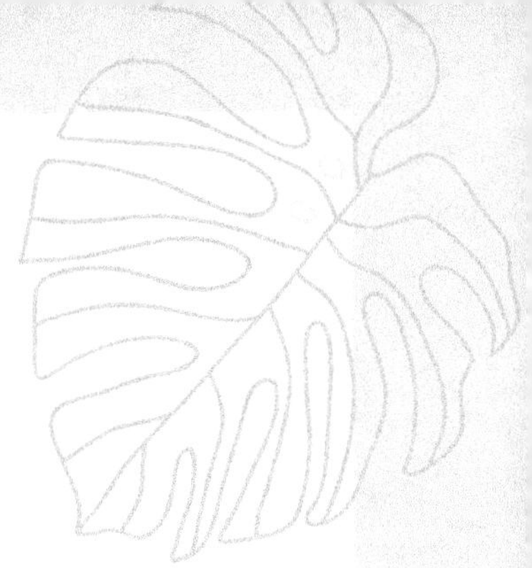

" You are never too old to transform.

The mind-body connection is powerful, and through yoga, you can cultivate a sense of calm and inner peace. Remember, practicing yoga is a gift to yourself.

Embrace it with joy, gratitude, and an open heart.

Namastè."

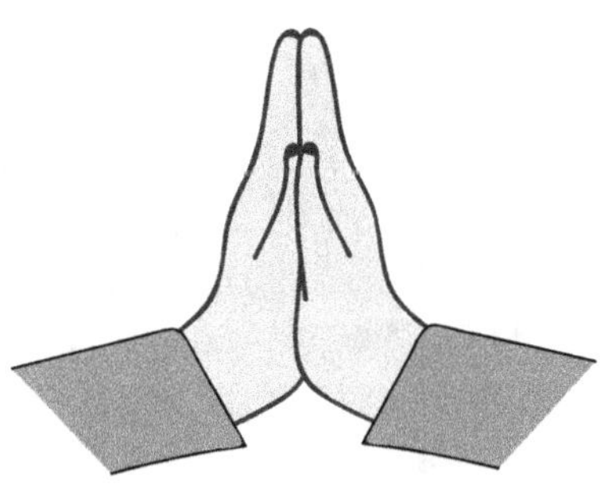

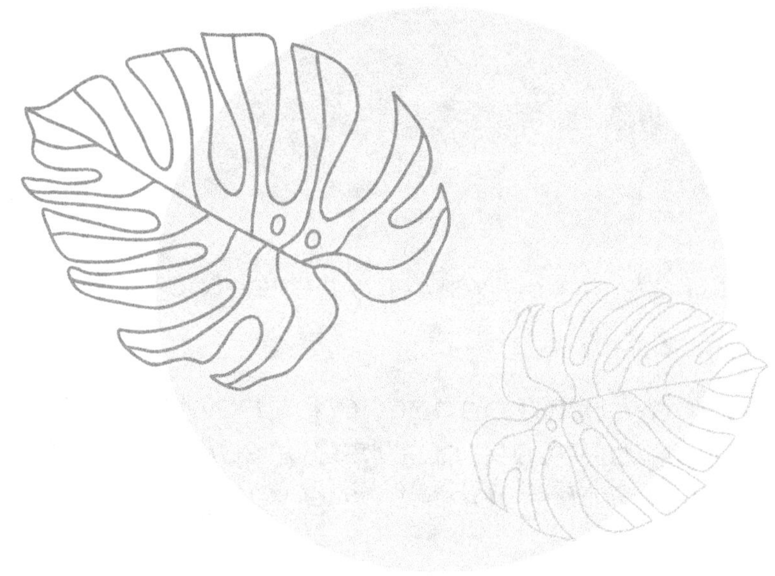